HEAVY
METAL

Out in the cold night
Our children wanders around
Why don't they understand?
Why don't they listen for a while?
You throw your lives away
With a petrol can today.
Please, please listen to what I say.

Hey you, only you kids
The future's in your hands
You can't put no faith
In the petrol in the can
You throw your lives away
With a petrol can today
Please, please listen to what I say

('Petrol Sniffing' by the Wedgetail Eagle Band,
Imparja Records, reproduced with kind permission of Victor Tunkin)

MAGGIE BRADY

HEAVY METAL

THE SOCIAL MEANING OF PETROL SNIFFING IN AUSTRALIA

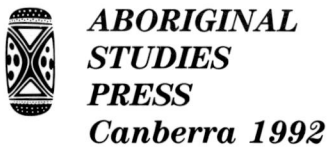

ABORIGINAL STUDIES PRESS
Canberra 1992

FIRST PUBLISHED IN 1992 BY
>Aboriginal Studies Press
>for the Australian Institute of Aboriginal and Torres Strait Islander Studies
>GPO Box 553, Canberra ACT 2601

>The views expressed in this publication are those of the author and not necessarily those of the Australian Institute of Aboriginal and Torres Strait Islander Studies.

© *MAGGIE BRADY 1992.*
>Apart from any fair dealing for the purpose of private study, research, criticism or review, as permitted under the Copyright Act, no part of this publication may be reproduced by any process whatsoever without the written permission of the publisher.

NATIONAL LIBRARY OF AUSTRALIA CATALOGUING-IN-PUBLICATION DATA:
>Brady, Maggie.
>Heavy metal: the social meaning of petrol sniffing in Australia.
>
>Includes index.
>Bibliography.
>ISBN 0 85575 215 7.
>
>[1]. Petrol sniffing — Australia. [2.] Aborigines, Australian — Substance abuse. 3. Solvent abuse — Australia. [4.] Aborigines, Australian — Health and hygiene. I. Title.
>
>362.299

>*TYPESET* in 9/14 Compugraphic Century Schoolbook by Jackie Covington, Aboriginal Studies Press
>*DESIGNED BY* Aboriginal Studies Press
>*COVER DESIGN BY* Denis French, Aboriginal Studies Press
>*PRINTED* on 115gsm semi matt by Southwood Press, Marrickville, New South Wales.
>*FRONT COVER* Caged petrol bowsers in Western Australia, 1988 (photograph by Maggie Brady)

3000 05 92

DEDICATION

To my mother 'Johnnie' Brady
and in memory of Jim Brady

CONTENTS

Illustrations	ix
Acknowledgements	xi
INTRODUCTION	1
The Drug, the Set and the Setting	3
The Research Methodology	5
Summary	7
CHAPTER 1 **AN OVERVIEW OF ABORIGINAL SUBSTANCE USE**	9
Populations and Substances of Choice	9
The Youthful Population	11
Defining the Problem	13
CHAPTER 2 **PATTERNS OF USE**	19
Studies of Cultural Differences between Indigenous Groups	19
Studies of Regional Variation Overseas	22
Regional Variation in Australia	27
CHAPTER 3 **SO TOXIC A SUBSTANCE**	37
The Toxicity of Petrol	37
Lead Absorption	38
Hydrocarbon Toxicity	39
Encephalopathy	40
Recovery	44
Clinic and Hospital Treatment	46
Chelation Therapy in Australia	47
CHAPTER 4 **THROWING THEIR LIVES AWAY**	53
Data on Aboriginal Deaths	53
The Distribution of Deaths in Australia	59
Susceptibility: The Role of Nutrition and Health Status	62
Evacuation and Treatment of Sniffers	64
CHAPTER 5 **STATEMENTS OF AUTONOMY**	69
Explanations as Strategies	69
Autonomy and Relatedness	72
My Body, My Business	75
'Getting Skinny': Anorexia and Petrol Sniffers	78
Commencing and Maintaining Use	82
Gangs and Heavy Metal	87
Refusing Incorporation	95

CHAPTER 6	**SANCTIONS**	99
	Informal Local Sanctions	100
	Socio-cultural Influences	102
	Access to Resources	111
	The Role of Christianity	113
	From Anglicans to Action	114
	Puritanical Influence in the Western Desert	119
	The Criminalisation of Petrol Sniffing	121
	Policing	129
	'The Welfare'	131
	Local Initiatives	132
	Social Restraints	134
CHAPTER 7	**THE SPREAD OF THE PRACTICE**	139
	The History of Petrol Sniffing	139
	Northern Australia	139
	Central Australia	146
	The Progression	150
	Presence and Absence of Petrol Sniffing	152
	Community Action	160
CHAPTER 8	**ACTION AND RESISTANCE**	169
	Social Meanings	169
	Social Actions	173
	Overseas Interventions	180
	The Influence of the Cattle Industry	183
CONCLUSION		191
REFERENCES		195
INDEX		217

ILLUSTRATIONS

FIGURES

1. Communities reporting petrol sniffing, New South Wales, to 1985 — 29
2. Communities reporting petrol sniffing, Queensland, to 1985 — 30
3. Communities reporting petrol sniffing, South Australia, to 1985 — 31
4. Communities reporting petrol sniffing, Western Australia, to 1985 — 32
5. Communities reporting petrol sniffing, Northern Territory, to 1985 — 33
6. Petrol-sniffing mortality by year, 1980–88 — 58
7. Petrol-sniffing mortality by month of death, 1980–88 — 59
8. Distribution of deaths associated with petrol sniffing, 1980–88 — 60
9. Evacuations to hospital from Maningrida for petrol-sniffing symptoms, 1984–88 — 65
10. Genealogy of the G____ family (Whitesand) and the M____ family (Blacksand) — 109
11. Anangu Pitjantjatjara Lands — 124
12. Communities reporting their first instance of petrol sniffing up to the present — 143
13. Distribution of marriage alliances, Pitjantjatjara region — 148
14. Routes by which petrol sniffing was disseminated — 153
15. Distribution of Central Australian languages — 155
16. Major Aboriginal communities, Arnhem Land — 159
17. Distribution of Kriol speakers — 163

PLATES

Unless otherwise indicated, photographs were taken by Maggie Brady.

1. Caged bowsers at a roadhouse in Western Australia — 13
2. An unsecured bowser, Arnhem Land — 16
3. Graffiti in Arnhem Land — 61
4. *Sniffer*, 1986, by Lin Onus — 71
5. Poster by Vanessa Nampijinpa Brown, 1984 — 76
6. Mad Dog Gang graffiti, east Arnhem Land — 88
7. Graffiti on school doors, east Arnhem Land — 90

8.	Rock musician, east Arnhem Land	92
9.	The Spit Gang graffiti, north-central Arnhem Land	92
10.	Rock gospel performance, east Arnhem Land	116
11.	Informal Christian music session, north-central Arnhem Land	117
12.	Ernabella central mission compound, 1966 (photograph Bill Edwards)	149

TABLES

1.	Aboriginal and Torres Strait Islander youth age groups by sex	10
2.	Aboriginal communities reporting petrol sniffing in 1985 and Aborigines as a percentage of the population by state	28
3.	Hospital treatment and outcome in eight cases of petrol-related encephalopathy	41
4.	Deaths caused by petrol sniffing in New Zealand, 1977–86	53
5.	Documented deaths caused by petrol sniffing among Aborigines, 1980–88	55
6.	Deaths caused by petrol sniffing by age, 1980–88	58
7.	Hospital evacuations by individual and sex, Maningrida, 1984–88	64
8.	Deaths caused by volatile substances by age, 1980–88	67
9.	Juvenile offences associated with substance abuse, 1986–89	127
10.	Petrol-sniffing related offences by age and sex, 1986–89	127
11.	Petrol-sniffing related offences, from most to least serious, and by age and sex, 1986–89	128

ACKNOWLEDGEMENTS

A great many individuals and organisations have unstintingly provided me with assistance while I was undertaking the fieldwork for the research reported here. It is simply not possible to name them all. I would like to thank the Research into Drug Abuse Advisory Committee of the Commonwealth Department of Community Services and Health, for the funding which made the research possible. The Principal of the Australian Institute of Aboriginal and Torres Strait Islander Studies willingly agreed to administer the grant and provided me with a base from which to work and the facilities of the Institute. Tibor Varga from the Institute was an exceptionally helpful Finance Officer. My colleagues in the research section gave me enthusiastic personal encouragement and professional support throughout the study, expecially Mary Edmunds, Kevin Keeffe and Debbie Rose.

I offer my grateful thanks to the following individuals and organisations; many of these people were generous with their hospitality in the bush, as well as offering their professional help.

In the Northern Territory: the Drug and Alcohol Bureau, Gordon Symons Centre, Healthy Aboriginal Life Team, Maningrida Council, the Menzies School of Health Research, the Ngaanyatjarra Council, Nganampa Health Council, the Pitjantjatjara Council, Central Australian Aboriginal Congress, Tangentyere Council, the Education Department, Vicky Burbank, Chris Connor, D Devaneson, David Daniels, Gayle Duell, Geoff Hanna, Richard Geeves, Grayson Gerrard, Rev Michael Gumbili, Greg Jarvis, Dinah Joshua, Lindsay Joshua, Trish Joy, Rob Moodie, Samuel Numamurdidi, Yulki Nunggumadjbar, Bobby Nunggumadjbar and Angurugu Local Government Council, Peter Oakes, Liz O'Neill, Glendle Schrader, Peter Tait, Maureen Tehan, Kaisu Vartto and Jo White.

In Western Australia: the Holyoake Institute, the Alcohol and Drug Authority, Rob Sheldon, Bill Genat, Duncan Graham, Jesse Habel, Linda Hayward, Liz McCullheh, David Martin, Damien McLean, Kevin Puertollano, Daire Phillips, Grace Richards, Terry Robinson, Steve Slocombe, Robin Smythe and Murray Wells. I am particularly indebted to Marian Kickett who enabled me to see the activities of the Working Party on Petrol Sniffing in the field, and helped in numerous other ways.

In South Australia: the Drug and Alcohol Services Council, Yalata Council, Richard Aspinall, Alice Cox, Brian Hobbs and the Aboriginal Health Organisation, George Koteka, Darcy O'Shea, Mabel Queama, Rene Sandimar and Trish Jenner.

In Canberra: the Alcohol and Drug Foundation Australia, Alf Leslie, David McDonald and Bill Wilson.

In 1990 I visited Canada as a World Health Organisation Fellow and held valuable discussions with Milton Tenenbein of the Winnipeg Children's

Hospital; Louis Fornazzari of the Clarke Institute of Psychiatry in Toronto; Randy Councillor of the Native Healers' Group in Kenora, Ontario; and Jill Torrie in Toronto. To these individuals I am particularly grateful.

I offer special thanks to the many friends and colleagues who have willingly shared their ideas and insights into drug use with me over the years, particularly Ross Kalucy, Pamela Lyon, Jan Reid, Carol Watson and Pamela Watson. Rodney Morice was instrumental in my initial involvement with research into petrol sniffing and Kingsley Palmer has supported my research with generosity and patience. I thank Sue Davenport (Research Assistant) and Jill Ross (who typed the manuscript) and anonymous reviewers for their comments; any errors remain my own.

INTRODUCTION

Drug use in our society is often interpreted as a solution to individually experienced pressures and strains. It is perceived, on the whole, to arise primarily out of individual psychopathology; that is, users and abusers are understood to be propelled into drug use by a variety of personal and interpersonal factors. These include dysfunctional or 'broken' families, low self-esteem, addictive personalities, psychological distress and the influence of friends. Drug use does not appear to be the prerogative of any particular section of society, and several writers on drug use have taken an historical and sociological approach, reminding us that, while the working classes of Mayhew's England used gin, the educated and privileged of that era used ether and cocaine (Mayhew's commentaries on the nineteenth-century labouring classes constituted an early urban ethnography). Marijuana and cocaine use are widespread today among the so-called middle classes.

Nevertheless, a different set of criteria are proposed to explain the antecedent causes of Aboriginal drug use and abuse. These relate to dispossession, colonisation, low socio-economic status and rapid social change. These are all eminently social factors. In other words, in contrast to our understanding of drug abuse in Western society, the reasons for Aboriginal drug abuse are seen to be primarily external, imposed factors rather than *individual* traits.

In part, the historical and socio-political factors that are thought to precipitate Aboriginal people into the overuse of certain drug substances are stressed in order to avoid 'blaming the victim'. It is now untenable for white Australians to avoid a frank reappraisal of the past, and we must accept responsibility for the indignities to which Aboriginal people were, and still are, subjected. In this context it is logical to interpret overuse of drug substances and alcohol as being but one manifestation of a variety of responses to oppressive social conditions. This can mean that, in order to avoid blaming the victim with respect to drug use, the social, rather than the individual, aspects of use are emphasised.

This presents a potential problem. The overemphasis on external factors and the use of a socio-political framework to explain a social problem perpetuates, in effect, the 'victimisation' of Aborigines. They are understood to be the helpless victims, overwhelmed by oppressive social circumstances and the power of a dominant society. Some Aboriginal people have themselves begun to question the nature of this stereotyping. For example, Merv Gibson, from Hope Vale, Queensland, has criticised both anthropologists and Aborigines for creating and perpetuating the 'myth' that Aboriginal people abuse alcohol (and we could include other drugs) because they are the passive victims of colonisation and culture clash (Gibson 1987). He also suggests that a myth has been created of a sharing culture which ostensibly makes it impossible for Aborigines to say no to alcohol. He continues (1987, 5):

> It is time to stop interpreting alcoholism as some kind of helpless result of culture clash. Rather we should see it for what it is: that is — the deliberate distortion of tradition for the sake of fulfilling an individual physical desire for alcohol. It is time to stop portraying the contemporary…alcoholic as a passive victim of colonisation. Rather we must consider how he has actively created his own problems.

There is another conceptual framework which has the effect of absolving the victim from blame — the disease model. This model proposes that alcoholism is a specific disease to which some people are vulnerable, and that these vulnerable individuals develop the disease if they take up drinking. Although applied primarily to alcoholism, the disease model is gaining ground among those Aboriginal people who have heard of it, as an explanation for other drug use, including the use of petrol. The disease model, which goes hand-in-hand with the notion of addiction, is set, as Kohn (1987, 36) so elegantly puts it, 'within an epic of relapse and confession'. He continues:

> Addiction is seen as a permanent component of the soul. This perspective combines the venerable religious concept of original sin with ideas from science: the 'disease' of addiction is like a viral infection which hijacks the organism's DNA chains and thus changes its fundamental genetic character.

From this perspective a petrol sniffer, like an alcoholic, is understood to have a 'sickness' emanating from within. This idea dramatically individualises the problem, but simultaneously relieves the bearer of the problem of blame. Significantly, it also relieves society of blame — in this case, white Australian society with Aboriginal people in its midst. Should popular (or, indeed, para-professional) opinion extend the disease analogy to petrol sniffing, there is a danger that the stereotype of Aborigines as hopeless and helpless victims will become entrenched. Beauvais and LaBoeff (1985, 158), in a thoughtful analysis of interventions in drug and alcohol abuse in American Indian communities comment:

> The unfortunate thing about stereotypes is that if they are pervasive enough, those to whom they are applied also begin to believe in them. When the lack of personal responsibility is combined with a belief in the inevitability of alcoholism [and 'addiction' to petrol] there develops a sense of fatalism that may defy treatment efforts. This sense of futility is felt by communities as well as by individuals — thus there is an acceptance that alcoholism is inevitable, and possibly untreatable.

From this rather simplified sketch of the opposing explanations for the drug abuse of Aborigines and others, it is clear that both the socio-political model and the disease model may serve to perpetuate a sense of fatalism among Aboriginal people. More seriously, by de-emphasising personal control of and responsibility for abuse and by focussing on external causes, these models make interventions feasible only on a grand scale, for example, the eradication of all forms of overt and covert social oppression, or on the level of primarily medical intervention.

These, then, are some of the anomalous areas in the understanding of drug use in Australia. There are several divergent views of the social and individual preconditions necessary for the occurrence of drug use and, moreover, strangely enough, these precipitating factors are presented as being mutually exclusive. At this point a further element that has a bearing on the debate about Aboriginal drug use can be introduced. As enacted social and economic policy, self-management for Aboriginal people aims for the encouragement of self-reliance, management and decision-making, and some degree of economic autonomy for Aboriginal communities. Self-management, said Viner in 1978 (3443),

> requires that Aboriginals, as individuals and communities, be in a position to make the same kinds of decisions about their future as other Australians customarily make, and to accept responsibility for the results following from those decisions.

The government response to many social problems in Aboriginal communities (and I refer particularly to traditionally oriented communities in remote Australia), in keeping with declared policy, is to assert that Aboriginal people themselves should discover and carry out the solutions to these problems. In the case of the form of drug use which is the subject of this book, petrol sniffing, a Senate Select Committee concluded after months of deliberation that 'there was unanimous and undisputed agreement that actions in response to petrol sniffing should originate and be controlled by the Aboriginal people in affected communities' (Commonwealth of Australia 1985, 220). It went on, however, to say that 'a number of people noted that many communities did not want to "own" the problem, considered that it was a "white-fella" problem, or considered that it was anyone else's problem but their own'. There is a startling paradox here. If communities consider that petrol sniffing is not their problem, then how can they be expected to devise workable responses over which they have 'control'?

THE DRUG, THE SET AND THE SETTING

In order to avoid the pitfalls inherent in the search for unified 'causes' for drug abuse — some of which have been touched on above — we can examine a framework articulated by Norman Zinberg that provides a useful starting point.

Zinberg (1984) states that in order to understand what impels someone to use an illicit drug, and how that drug affects the user, three determinants must be considered: the drug (the pharmacological actions of the substance itself); the set (the attitude of the person at the time of use, including his or her personality structure); and the setting (the influence of the physical and social setting within which the use occurs).

Significantly, Zinberg suggests that, of the three variables, the setting has received the least attention and recognition. This may explain why so much of our present understanding of drug use in the general population is oriented towards individual psychopathology; the setting has indeed been neglected, and yet in some respects it is the most significant variable. Zinberg (1984, 14-15) continues:

> The social setting, with its formal and informal controls, its capacity to develop new informal social sanctions and rituals, and its transmission of information in numerous informal ways, is a crucial factor in the controlled use of any intoxicant. This does not mean that the pharmaceutical properties of the drug or the attitudes and personality of the user count for little or nothing. All three variables — drug, set and setting — must be included in any valid theory of drug use. It is necessary to understand in every case how the specific characteristics of the drug and the personality of the user interact and are modified by the social setting and its controls.

Although Zinberg derived this framework from a study of what he refers to as 'controlled' intoxicant use (ie drug users regulated their own intake), rather than what might be termed 'compulsive' intoxicant use (in which users were unable to control their intake), his framework provides a broad perspective which encompasses both individual and societal features. It is equally applicable as a means of understanding dysfunctional drug use, because it allows consideration of formal and informal controls and considers whether these exist at all.

Because it utilises the Zinberg model, this study devotes considerable attention to the setting in which young Aboriginal people sniff petrol and the interaction between set and setting. Initially, however, I provide an overview of the use of drug substances among Aboriginal people, and this review is contained in Chapter One. Chapter Two addresses the work published on the use of petrol as an inhalant among indigenous and minority groups overseas with particular emphasis on regional variation. Chapters Three and Four look at the substance itself: petrol and its toxic components and effects. In this respect petrol is not normally considered to be a drug substance; its functions lie primarily elsewhere. Chapter Five deals with the set: the individual user and groups of users, and the variety of subjective motivations that may be associated with the use of petrol. Chapter Six analyses the setting variables which influence the use of petrol, particularly social sanctions and difficulties with their implementation. Chapter Seven examines the genesis and subsequent dispersion of the practice of petrol sniffing, and analyses some anomalies in the distribution, looking in detail at some communities which have curbed the practice. The final chapter presents data from Australia and overseas that documents interventions and provides a hypothesis whereby we can explain the absence of the practice in particular regions.

THE RESEARCH METHODOLOGY

In the course of the research reported here, I undertook periods of fieldwork in the Northern Territory and Central and Western Australia. I had intended to spend some time in the far north of South Australia in the Pitjantjatjara Lands, but my request for permission to undertake research in those communities was not granted, as the Council felt that enough research had been undertaken on petrol sniffing. My work in Western Australia was undertaken with the assistance of, and in conjunction with, the State Working Party on Petrol Sniffing, coordinated by Marian Kickett. I spent time in Warburton, Blackstone, Jameson, Wingellina and Warakuna, and visited the region on three occasions. In the Northern Territory, I made research trips to Alice Springs, Tennant Creek and Ali Curung and spent two longer periods of fieldwork further north in Ngukurr, Numbulwar and Angurugu (Groote Eylandt). I made several visits to Darwin to meet with staff at the Royal Darwin Hospital, the Menzies School of Health Research, the Drug and Alcohol Bureau and the Gordon Symons Centre, and briefly visited Milingimbi and Galiwin'ku, with a longer trip to Maningrida at the request of the Northern Territory Health Department.

As I was interested in why some communities do not have petrol sniffers I visited some of these (Kununurra, Tennant Creek, Ali Curung and Ngukurr). It was particularly difficult to investigate the absence of sniffing in a community, because I was anxious that widespread community knowledge of my business might prompt an inordinate interest in the substance. People were naturally puzzled as to what I was doing there when they had no problem with petrol.

Overall the study was conducted, and is reported, primarily from an anthropological perspective rather than an epidemiological or medical one, although it is informed by these disciplines. The fieldwork visits involved a combination of participant observations and informal interviews with community members, community Council members and non-Aboriginal staff, particularly community health sisters at local clinics. In some cases, I drew upon my knowledge of the communities gained in previous years. Where feasible, I also collected statistical data on morbidity and mortality associated with petrol sniffing. Some Aboriginal medical services have now begun to collect statistics by providing a category for petrol and alcohol-related presentations on their printed daily record sheets completed in clinics. The collection of statistical data was not easy, as surprisingly little formal data collection is undertaken on sniffing as a matter of course. Evacuations from their home communities to a town-based hospital of patients suffering from symptoms related to sniffing are often entered in individual community clinic records, but are not collated according to diagnosis by regional aerial medical services. Case histories of petrol sniffers are kept on their personal medical files: no communities keep ongoing records on petrol sniffers unless they employ a community worker who is working specifically with young people. Police departments and local police stations, schools in Aboriginal communities and even federal and state governments (with some exceptions) collect little or no data on petrol sniffing. Despite government agencies' sporadic attempts to combine the observations and knowledge of their regional representatives, this has rarely resulted in any formal ongoing collection of information.

I did not use questionnaires or any formal surveys, although I tried to collect basic data on each community. I considered that questionnaires would have been problematic, particularly in schools, as they probably would have directed attention at petrol sniffing in a counterproductive way. I utilised available sources of statistical information on each community, including population data from the Australian Bureau of Statistics and the community profiles on 'community problems' from the Statistics Unit of the Department of Aboriginal Affairs. To a large extent, I pursued a rigorous line of inquiry in the field, while also participating in informal interactions with people. In this way, my initial hypotheses were tested, checked and found wanting in some cases. Several entirely unexpected areas of inquiry opened up in the latter part of my research, including one associated with the user's subjective decision to sniff petrol, and another associated with the mortality data. I also gathered data on particular communities and regions from ex-missionaries and their staff and from my anthropological colleagues who had undertaken long-term fieldwork in those areas.

As the Pitjantjatjara experience shows, gaining permission from Aboriginal organisations and communities to undertake research into this issue has not been easy. Communities are sensitive about researchers in general, and petrol sniffing in particular, and the main reason for this is that the many brief and often superficial investigative visits or quick surveys (mainly by government departments) that have occurred have attracted unwelcome media attention. As a result of this interest, Aboriginal communities now have the mistaken impression that a considerable amount of 'research' has been done into sniffing, which is not the case. It has been necessary to use the names of communities concerned (which are, in any case, already public as a result of the report of the Senate Select Committee on Volatile Substance Fumes in Australia), but in other cases I have avoided identifying specific locations.

It was disturbing to discover that there are very few resources made available to communities on the subject; that there is a great deal of misinformation among Aboriginal and non-Aboriginal community members about the effects of petrol sniffing; and that there is an absence of medical protocols and guidelines for community clinics to follow when dealing with affected individuals. Government departments have only recently sorted out who is 'responsible' for petrol-sniffing related issues, and their approaches still lack coordination and direction. Communities are still confused about where they should apply for funds or where to seek advice.

SUMMARY

Petrol sniffing, during which the volatile hydrocarbons emitted by petrol are deliberately inhaled in order to achieve alteration in mood, is but one of a variety of abuses of volatile substances. Most of the petrol inhaled in the regions under consideration is leaded petrol, and chronic sniffers thus suffer the physical consequences associated with the toxic components in the volatile hydrocarbons, as well as the toxic heavy metal, lead, contained in petrol. Sniffers are young adult and adolescent Aborigines, usually between the ages of ten and twenty-five, living predominantly in two Australian states (Western Australia and South Australia) and the Northern Territory. In these three regions the total Aboriginal population between the ages of ten and twenty-four is 30,548, according to the 1986 Census (South Australia: 4,896; Western Australia: 13,435; Northern Territory: 12,217). A very approximate estimation of the number of chronic petrol sniffers in South Australia, Western Australia and the Northern Territory, which includes known habitual, rather than occasional, users, is between 600 and 1,000. This means that bewween 2 and 3 per cent of Aborigines in the ten to twenty-four age group in the Northern Territory, Western Australia and South Australia regularly use petrol at present. I stress that these are approximations and that fluctuations are constantly occurring. Nevertheless, this estimate shows that a very small proportion of this age group engages in the practice, an important fact to bear in mind while reading this book.

CHAPTER

1 AN OVERVIEW OF ABORIGINAL SUBSTANCE USE

POPULATIONS AND SUBSTANCES OF CHOICE

The Australian population, like many Western societies, most commonly uses and abuses legal drugs, particularly alcohol and tobacco, and these drugs are associated with more chronic illness, disease, accidents, social problems and days off work than all the other drugs put together (Brown et al 1986, 73; Drew 1983). Approximately 80 per cent of adult Australians use alcohol and 10 per cent of adults aged twenty-five to sixty-four years are regarded as being at risk because they regularly consume more than five drinks a day (Brown et al 1986). Total adult consumption of alcohol across all ages is highest in the Northern Territory and lowest in South Australia (Commonwealth of Australia 1988).

Aboriginal people in Australia also mainly use the legal drugs: alcohol, tobacco, analgesics, solvents and kava, although there are some unofficial reports that note the use of illegal drugs among urban Aborigines.[1] In remote areas, restricted availability narrows the range of substances used. Nevertheless alcohol, tobacco, inhalants (particularly petrol), kava, and methanol are often available, even in bush communities.

The 1986 Census of Population and Housing estimated the Aboriginal and Islander population to be 227,645, 1.4 per cent of the total Australian population. The figure included Aborigines who live what is often termed a 'traditional' life, practise their religious Law and long-established economic activities, as well as people who live in rural towns and urban centres. Indeed a majority of the Aboriginal population (66 per cent) resides in urban or semi-urban areas. The 83,427 young Aborigines between the ages of ten and twenty-four make up 37 per cent of the total Aboriginal population (see Table 1).

Most research and social welfare attention concerning Aboriginal drug abuse has been focussed on alcohol — a drug long thought to be about to precipitate the demise of the race. This view is still held by some researchers today (see Spencer 1988). Tobacco and alcohol are the mood-altering substances most commomly used by Aboriginal people today and, although the assumption that alcohol abuse would destroy Aboriginal society has proved incorrect, it is hard to deny that this practice causes high rates of morbidity, premature death and acute social distress among Aboriginal populations. Since there is no nationwide system for the separate identification of Aboriginal deaths in death registration statistics, information on

Aboriginal mortality rates (with respect to alcohol or any other cause) remains fragmented (Plant 1988). It is possible to glean some information on Aboriginal mortality and morbidity associated with alcohol from individual states and territories (see Hunt 1981; Thomson 1985; Devanesen et al 1986; Plant 1988).

An indication of the social stresses associated with alcohol abuse is to be found in studies by social scientists, particularly anthropologists (see Bain 1974; Beckett 1965; Barber et al 1988; Brady and Palmer 1984; Collmann 1988; O'Connor 1984; Sansom 1980). In recent years, Aboriginal organisations have undertaken their own research into alcohol abuse, in order to make submissions to government bodies. Government-sponsored inquiries have progressed from the rather general Parliamentary Standing Committee investigations to more specific, in-depth investigations of particular areas, the impact of alcohol upon populations and their liquor control requirements (see Northern Territory Liquor Commission 1982; Hedges 1986; D'Abbs 1987; Legislative Assembly of the Northern Territory 1991).

Tobacco use, in the form of smoking and tobacco chewing, is widespread in the Aboriginal population. A Northern Territory survey of drug use patterns in Aboriginal communities found that over half of those interviewed smoked, and one-quarter chewed tobacco (Watson et al 1988). In different regions of the country Aboriginal people smoke cigarettes, varieties of pipes, and chew tobacco mixed with the ash of particular species of trees. Tobacco use was entrenched in Aboriginal social life before the arrival of Europeans two hundred years ago, with the use of indigenous *Nicotiana* plants as well as imported tobaccos brought by

Table 1: Aboriginal and Torres Strait Islander youth age groups by sex, ages 10–24

Ages	10–14	15–19	20–24	Total
Males	15,517	14,475	11,847	41,839
Females	14,760	14,631	12,197	41,588
Total	30,277	29,106	24,044	83,427

Total Aboriginal and TSI population in Australia: 227,645
Aborigines and TSI youth (aged 10–24): 83,427 (37% of total)

(Source: ABS and John Done, Statistics Section, Department of Aboriginal Affairs *Community Profiles*, 1985)

Indonesian sailors (Macknight 1976; Thomson 1939). Thomson believed that Aboriginal people were already addicted to their indigenous tobacco, so that the regular supplies of 'stick' tobacco, which accompanied white settlement, found a ready clientele. The two leading causes of death among Northern Territory Aborigines are circulatory and respiratory diseases: both are associated with smoking (Watson et al 1988).

Analgesic use was found to be widespread and frequent among Aborigines living in rural New South Wales in the 1970s (Kamien 1975) and more recently, Watson et al (1988) found the use of 'tablets' (including analgesics and benzodiazepines) widespread among the Northern Territory Aborigines interviewed.[2]

Kava (made from the root of the pepper plant *Piper methysticum*) is legally imported into Australia as a food beverage not a drug, and since 1982 has become popular in at least six communities in coastal regions of the Northern Territory (Alexander et al 1987). In July 1988 Western Australia restricted access to kava by invoking Section 22 of the Poisons Act 1964, so that its use is now legal only with a permit. The pharmacological actions of kava are as a local anaesthetic, a centrally acting muscle relaxant and as a sedative. These effects are considered by Aboriginal users to make kava a preferable alternative to alcohol. Despite the fact that kava is widely used in the southwestern Pacific and is believed to be harmless if taken in moderation with a balanced diet, Mathews et al (1988) found in a pilot study that heavy users of kava were underweight, complained of poor health and might be experiencing some liver damage.

THE YOUTHFUL POPULATION

The use of petrol as an inhalant dominates the published accounts of substance use by young Aborigines, although some data is available on the use of other substances. In 1986 a survey of Aboriginal school students in New South Wales was published (New South Wales Aboriginal Education Consultative Group 1986) which questioned 272 students, adopting a non-threatening approach by asking for information based on their knowledge of drug and alcohol use by other young people, rather than their own use. The survey asked about the use of alcohol, tobacco, inhaled substances and other drugs (marijuana, tranquillisers, cocaine and heroin). Ninety per cent of the students knew other young Aborigines who drank beer, while 30 per cent admitted that they smoked (the smoking question was directed to the respondent). Forty per cent of the students knew others who sniffed petrol and slightly fewer knew glue sniffers.

The Northern Territory survey (Watson et al 1988) found that alcohol was used by 36.6 per cent of young Aborigines in the fifteen to twenty age group and by 48 per cent of the twenty-one to thirty age group. In both groups there were substantially more male than female users. On Palm Island in Queensland, researchers noted that children sometimes stole beer from the licensed canteen, and liquor offences there included the supply of alcohol to minors (Barber et al 1988). However, in many regions there are strong informal rules which discourage the use of alcohol by young adolescents (Brady and Palmer 1984), and drinking by those considered to be too young provokes argument and punishment.

There has been little research undertaken so far into the use of tobacco by young Aboriginal people, although the Northern Territory survey found that smoking was usually a well-established practice by the age of twenty years (Watson et al 1988). There are considerable regional and gender differences in the use of tobacco; for example, chewing tobacco is more common among desert Aborigines and among women than among northern groups. In Ngaanyatjarra-speaking communities in Western Australia I have observed young girls six or seven years old chewing tobacco.

For reasons of availability, cheapness and lack of access to other substances, the inhalation of volatile substances is particularly appealing to young Aborigines, as it is to non-Aboriginal youth, both in Australia and elsewhere. In New South Wales 42 per cent of the Aboriginal schoolchildren surveyed knew between one and ten other young people using glue, petrol, thinner or spray cans as inhalants, and 8 per cent knew someone younger than nine years of age inhaling such substances (New South Wales Aboriginal Education Consultative Group, 1986). Anecdotal reports in the press have referred to young urban Aborigines using inhalants, and in urban gaols the inhalation of volatile solvents is just one of a number of drug uses practised (see *West Australian* 22 December 1987; *Canberra Times* 2 July 1988). After reports of Aboriginal children sniffing glue in Brisbane, the Queensland government proposed new laws to search for and detain children suffering from the effects of inhaled substances (*National Times* 12 December 1981; Robson 1982). The Senate Select Committee into Volatile Substance Fumes reported that 'glue sniffing' occurred in inner-city areas of Brisbane in 1980 with the majority of public users being Aborigines (Commonwealth of Australia 1985, 26–27). The committee compiled a summary of known mortality in each state as a result of volatile substance use (Commonwealth of Australia 1985, 38).

The use of deliberately inhaled volatile substances, specifically petrol, is more prevalent in remote Aboriginal communities than in urban or rural populations. The former are usually smaller populations of up to 1,000 people residing in settlements which function as incorporated Aboriginal communities, and which were once run by missions or other welfare agencies. This category also includes town camps, fringe camps and people living on small portions of land excised from freehold or leasehold land. In addition, there are small groups of Aboriginal people living in outstations or homeland centres, decentralised communities which have split away from longer-established settlements. There are three regions where petrol sniffing is most prevalent: western, central and eastern Arnhem Land in the Northern Territory; Central Australia including the regions bordering South Australia, Western Australia and the Northern Territory; and the Eastern Goldfields region of Western Australia.

DEFINING THE PROBLEM

> Heavy inhalant users...[are] a population which may have impact beyond their numbers (Carroll 1977, 17).

It is hard to withstand the temptation to refer to petrol sniffing, unthinkingly, as a 'problem', when this is the orientation of the majority of written and spoken comment on the practice. Government agencies responsible for the health and well-being of Aboriginal people have only recently come to believe that petrol sniffing is a serious drug-use problem, although it has been many years since the issue came to prominence through the first published research into the practice (Nurcombe et al 1970), and through a flurry of newspaper reports which appeared

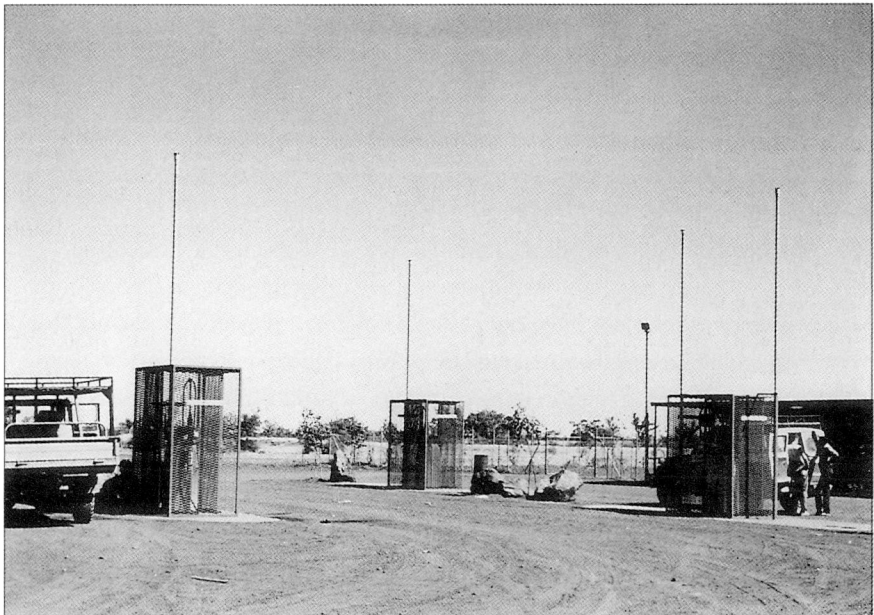

Plate 1: Caged bowsers at a roadhouse in Western Australia

in the late 1970s and early 1980s. In 1983 a Northern Territory senator called for the establishment of a Senate Select Committee to inquire into 'petrol and glue sniffing' in Australia (*Centralian Advocate* 25 November 1983). The Senate Select Committee on Volatile Substance Fumes was duly convened, made its inquiries and reported in December 1985. It nominated three broad reasons why Aboriginal petrol sniffing was a problem (Commonwealth of Australia 1985):

1. the severe physical and psychological effects on those involved;
2. the impact of sniffing on a fragile social system such that it threatens to destroy it completely;
3. the extent and considerable magnitude of the problem.

It is important, however, to remind ourselves that different cultures may hold very different views about what constitutes a drug use problem and why. The perspective apparent in many government reports on the subject is not entirely free of ideological overtones. For example, sniffers are often referred to as 'itinerant' (Commonwealth of Australia 1985, 27), a demeaning term used to refer to gipsies and 'undesirables' elsewhere, people who, for the very reason that they have no settled place of abode, are deemed to be marginal and thus threatening to those with a proper sense of 'place' (Foucault 1979).

Petrol sniffing by young people, often in groups, constitutes a threat, both physically and metaphorically, to the social order. For a long time the incidence of petrol sniffing has been gauged 'more by the degree of social disruption and damage to property...than by the actual incidence or extent of petrol inhalation' (Hayward-Ryan 1979, 1). Drug use of this variety appears to threaten some states more than others. Sniffing by young Aborigines in Queensland, for example, was seen to provide 'an opportunity for those children from depressed environments to blatantly incite society. This flaunting of authority appears to be an integral part of Aboriginal glue sniffing' (Commonwealth of Australia 1985, 26).

Young Aborigines who use petrol are often depicted as having nothing to do, as coming from deprived homes, as being unemployed and playing truant from school. Solutions involving meaningful employment are often mooted. Concerns such as these reinforce the comment by Kohn (1987) that implicit in the social struggle over drug use are the virtues of thrift, temperance, industry and family responsibility. Constant employment has long been seen as a remedy for the 'erring poor'. The significance of the focus on juveniles (often undeserved) is that it deflects attention from adult deviance. Even when the activities of juvenile Aboriginal sniffers are said to 'threaten' indigenous customary rules rather than the social order of the dominant society, it is rarely acknowledged that these rules are violated by many other members of that society. Calling the names of the dead, for example, said to be a deliberate breach of traditional codes of conduct by sniffers, is a common feature of the drunken comportment of adults. Similarly, the sexual exploits which may undermine marriage plans transacted by adults for young people are indulged in by Aboriginal people (as by all human societies) whether influenced by alcohol, drugs or no substance use at all. These examples were both cited in the Senate Select Committee report.

We are mistaken if we assume that the members of any society inevitably and unfailingly observe the social rules. As Jaffe observes (1983, 106) in a discussion of different cultural definitions of drug problems, 'since in most societies sinners outweigh the saints by a goodly margin, it is not always clear why the sins of drug use are singled out for special condemnation'. Perhaps the answer rests, at least in part, in the notion that by making a fuss about drugs, society creates channels for the discharge of anxieties larger than the drug issue itself would merit (Kohn 1987). Drug use has been portrayed in the past as being a 'threat' to entire nations and both alcohol and petrol sniffing are now posited as threatening the 'extinction' of the race (Spencer 1988, 20) and the destruction of the 'fragile social system' of Aborigines (Commonwealth of Australia 1985, 161). Although drug taking, particularly heavy alcohol consumption, may cause untold misery, there is little historical evidence of whole societies being destroyed by drugs. In opposition to the idea that drug abuse will somehow lay the body politic low from within, Kohn (1987, 28) states that: 'In fact, societies seem to display an extraordinary resilience in the face of mass intoxication: it is individuals who do not'.

Together with the perpetuation of the myth of a 'golden age' in which young people unquestioningly obeyed the law and listened with respect to their elders, the idea that drug use is about to destroy a society (in this case Aboriginal society) is something of a timeless phenomenon. As I have observed elsewhere, the ethnographers Spencer and Gillen heard complaints in 1899 from elderly Aborigines that the young people no longer cared for the traditions of their fathers. The grandsons of those errant youths undoubtedly make the same complaints today (Brady 1985a, 24; Pearson 1983). It is partly because of the myth that Aboriginal society was unchanging, that conflict was absent (particularly inter-generational conflict), and that drug use is 'new', that petrol sniffing is often discussed in terms of its threat to Aboriginal society. As Jaffe (1983, 105) notes, in many instances the origins of concern over use of a drug may,

> with the passage of time, become blurred and disconnected. A society begins to view the drug itself as a threat. From time to time we need to remind ourselves about why we are concerned so that we can direct our remedies to the sources of our concern.

Apart from the belief that petrol sniffing is a problem because it threatens the social fabric of Aboriginal life and that it manifestly disturbs the social order, sniffing is considered to be a serious health problem. This was the first conclusion of the Senate Select Committee. Although, as will be shown in this study, mortality and morbidity associated with petrol sniffing are not inconsiderable, it is nevertheless apparent that many forms of behaviour lead to impaired health and social functioning. Another significant aspect of the association between petrol sniffing and health is that large numbers of Aboriginal people have used petrol as an inhalant with little apparent ill effect. This fact has profound implications for health education as well as for Aboriginal perceptions of the dangers of the practice.

So far I have dealt primarily with the concerns of non-Aboriginal Australians about the drug use of Aboriginal Australians. But do Aboriginal people see sniffing as a problem? At the level of what might be termed official discourse, community councils, chairpersons, health workers and other spokespeople express alarm about sniffing and demand assistance with solutions. But large numbers

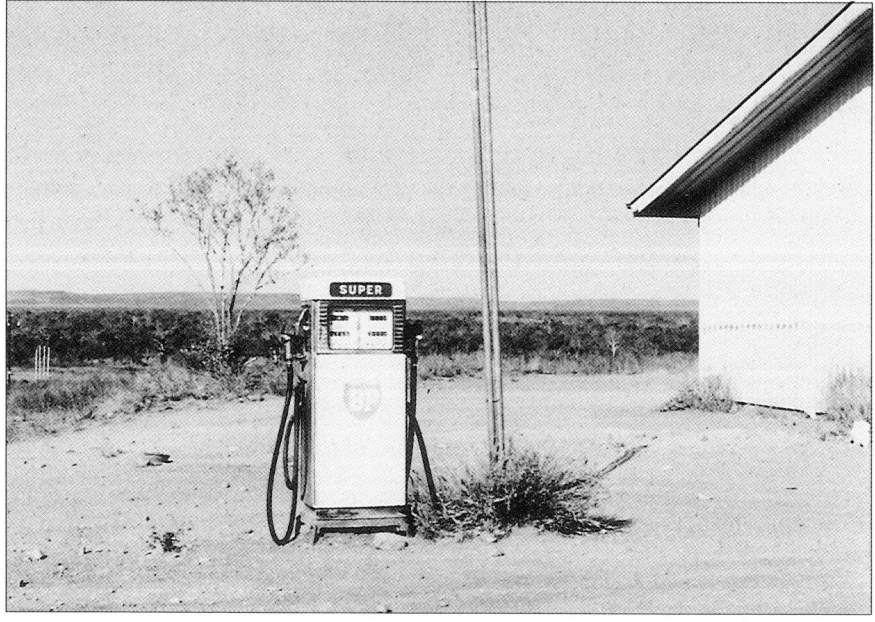

Plate 2: An unsecured bowser in an Arnhem Land settlement which has curbed petrol sniffing

of Aboriginal people have succeeded in living with and accommodating petrol sniffing, which makes abstract problem-definition more difficult. Sniffers are part of the human geography of life in bush communities. When a sniffer has seizures or becomes unconscious, someone seeks help from the nursing sister. The sniffer is placed in the clinic, receives sedatives, is visited by concerned relatives, perhaps is evacuated to a city hospital. Later the sniffer returns, rather tremulous and unsteady on his or her feet, but improved, and is received back into his or her family. A local welfare worker (Elsegood nd, 6) wrote of Maningrida some years ago:

> I am of the opinion most parents do not see sniffing as a problem, except in those areas where it brings them into conflict with authority. The attempts to eradicate petrol sniffing have always been instigated, and in most cases carried out by European authority figures, eg police, health, education and welfare... . With Aboriginal people who try and get them to take action, parents are much more aggressive and are inclined to tell them to mind their own business or threaten them with violence.

Since this was written, interventions (involving education, raised community awareness and direct action) instigated and supported by Aboriginal people themselves are now more prevalent. The Healthy Aboriginal Life Team (HALT) in Central Australia has adopted interventions which involve direct counselling of users and their families, and which utilise paintings and posters to explain the spread of sniffing and to increase awareness. The Western Australian government established a coordinating Working Party on Petrol Sniffing, which has taken a consciousness-raising approach, giving workshops in Aboriginal settlements and encouraging local initiatives. This group's approach emphasises raising the esteem of remote settlement dwellers with the aim of empowering communities so that action can occur. Funding has been made available to some communities for diversionary activities; some regions have local by-laws in place which mean that the police may apprehend sniffers and refer them to other agencies. Despite these developments, communities in which sniffing has become an entrenched practice (over a matter of some twenty years) still evince a level of weary tolerance for the practice which makes determined action almost impossible. Elsegood's comments noted above are still apposite today in certain areas. The factors which influence a tolerant attitude towards petrol sniffing, and those which have the unintentional effect of undermining local initiatives, are examined later in this study. In short, it is not possible to provide an unequivocal answer to the question of whether Aboriginal people define petrol sniffing to be a problem. The gap between official representations and the lived reality is, at times, revealing.

NOTES

1. For example, marijuana use was reported in Lockridge, Western Australia (*Sunday Times* 1 November 1987); heroin use in Wellington, New South Wales (*Daily Telegraph* 29 July 1988).

2. As I have documented elsewhere, Aboriginal people not only knew how to make apparently intoxicating beverages in pre-contact times, they had access to a variety of mood-altering substances including *pituri* and soporific drugs (Brady 1985a; Watson 1983; Carr and Carr 1981). The only accounts of inhaled substances other than smoke from tobacco pipes refer to the inhalation of smoke from acacia leaves in order to calm overexcited children on Groote Eylandt, Northern Territory (Levitt 1981), and the inhalation of the perfume and perhaps the pollen of wattle blossoms 'used as an opiate to cause sleep' by Tasmanian Aborigines (Plomley 1966). Kava, widely understood to be a substance 'new' to Australia, was drunk by Torres Strait Islanders early this century, according to a first-hand account by a resident teacher (Chief Protector of Aborigines *Annual Report* 1911).

CHAPTER

PATTERNS OF USE

The question of regional and socio-cultural variations in drug use has been addressed by only a few anthropologically oriented studies, most of them from overseas. Such studies are important because they call into question stereotypes that depict indigenous or minority groups as substance abusers en masse, and as being homogenous populations who have responded similarly to the historical and political stresses placed upon them. The reality is that indigenous and minority populations are rarely homogenous, and have resorted to substance abuse in varying degrees and with diverse outcomes. In Australia, the Northern Territory Survey of Drug Use Patterns in Aboriginal Communities found striking variations between people in the tropical north and in Central Australia. These variations were found in the statistics on the frequency of drinking alcohol; the age at commencement of drinking; the methods of using tobacco; and in the choice of substances used. My own research has identified distinct regions where petrol sniffing is practised and others where it is not.

STUDIES OF CULTURAL DIFFERENCES BETWEEN INDIGENOUS GROUPS

Perhaps the greatest value of intra-group and inter-regional studies is that they question the notion of acculturation — the idea that social disorganisation among indigenous or minority groups has resulted from the 'clash' with modern Western society. The process of acculturation is said to be associated with stress resulting from value conflicts, identity crises and the loss of traditional institutions. Those thought to be most stressed by acculturation 'have been found to engage in maladaptive behaviours, including drug abuse' (Bonnheim and Korman 1985, 25). From this perspective there is a supposedly natural progression from groups who are firmly entrenched in their traditional ways — and therefore less likely to produce high levels of deviant behaviour — to those who are undergoing rapid social and cultural change, and are encroached upon by modernisation, and who exhibit high levels of deviance (May 1982, 1200). Thus Barnes asserts of petrol sniffing among native Canadian groups that 'heavy abuse occurs where cultural changes are occurring' (1985, 146). He cites Nurcombe's study of petrol sniffing at Galiwin'ku as evidence of this (Nurcombe et al 1970), but Nurcombe does not explain why petrol sniffing was not present among neighbouring groups who were also experiencing rapid cultural changes.

These assertions make several questionable assumptions, including the notion that non-acculturated (ie 'traditional') society was unchanging, and also that cultural change is necessarily stressful. Many would argue that Aboriginal people have in fact adopted Western technologies and value systems extremely successfully in some cases. Beauvais and LaBoeff (1985, 154) are more perceptive when they comment that

> most research has attempted to find differences between traditional and non-traditional groups of people. It is likely that the situation is more complex and involves an expanded classification...[there is a] third category [which is] not merely a halfway point between Indian and White culture.

One of the most significant anthropologically oriented studies of alcohol use among American Indian groups to date analysed the epidemiology of alcohol-related morbidity among two neighbouring tribes (Kunitz et al 1971). Ironically, in view of the above discussion on acculturation, Kunitz and his colleagues found a higher rate of alcohol-related cirrhosis (liver disease) among the more traditionally oriented of the two groups. The Hopi and the Navaho lived side-by-side in northern Arizona and had been subjected to similar external circumstances, but nevertheless showed significantly different rates of alcoholic cirrhosis. Consumption of alcohol was common among both groups. Drinking among the Navaho was highly visible and groups of young men leading a traditional pastoral life drank particularly excessively. However, the Navahos had a much lower rate of cirrhosis than the Hopi, the majority of whom lived in traditional villages where cultural values were firmly maintained, and where 'acting out' while drunk was disvalued as not being in keeping with the 'Hopi way' of peace and harmony. The researchers suggest that the high cirrhosis rate among Hopis was because heavy drinkers were ejected from the community as a result of collective disapproval. Devoid of social and community supports they continued to drink, and thus were more likely to develop cirrhosis. The Navaho on the other hand tended to be either abstainers or heavy drinkers as young men, but many of them stopped drinking before their health was affected. As a result of their findings, Kunitz and his colleagues questioned the assumption that 'acculturation stress' explains problem drinking, and suggested that there are many important cultural differences that exist between tribes (Kunitz et al 1971).

Another American social scientist has studied the prevalence and susceptibility of different American Indian populations to substance abuse (May 1982). Looking first at alcohol use among indigenous Americans, he observes that the prevalence varies widely from one reservation to the next. Comparing prevalence of use among these adults with the United States average, he found that the Ute and Ojibwa had higher levels of alcohol use than the national average. The Standing Rock Sioux were about the same, and one group was considerably lower than the United States average. Despite these differences all of them had reputations as 'hard drinking groups'. May also found variability based on tribal and/or geographic areas for the use of marijuana by American Indians, and higher overall rates of prevalence than the national average. The use of inhalants (including petrol, glue and solvents) is reported to be twice as high among Indians aged twelve to seventeen than the United States averages. May (1982, 1196) comments that more cross-tribal research on inhalant use is necessary. He goes on to suggest that there is a 'traditional cultural factor' which may explain differences in 'deviant' behaviour so that 'tribes which are characterised by loose, small-group or band-level organisation have been found to produce more individualistic behaviour which is now considered deviant behaviour'. He does not say whose definition of deviance this is, but continues,

> On the other hand, tribes which are organised in larger groups have a more rigid and fixed social structure, were historically and are contemporarily much more prone to produce deviance … . In this manner, traditional social organisation has been found to be important in producing or impeding deviance such as alcohol problems, suicide, crime, etc. Drug use should also follow this pattern to some degree.

Such a culturally deterministic analysis is interesting, and may indeed have some value, but it does not ask whose perception of deviance we are considering. Alcohol abuse and actions defined as 'crimes' may not be considered deviant within particular populations or sub-groups — a fact that theories of deviance first brought to prominence over fifty years ago. As Erikson wrote in 1962, 'Deviance is not a property *inherent* in certain forms of behaviour; it is a property *conferred upon* those forms by the audience which directly or indirectly witness them' (Erikson 1962, 308). Notwithstanding these caveats, May's suggestion that the nature of social organisation itself (rather than the presence or absence of 'traditional' mores) may influence the prevalence of 'deviant' behaviour is a useful contribution to the debate. It may not necessarily explain the aetiology of unsociable or deviant behaviour, but it does explain why some populations are able to introduce effective social controls and others are not.

Literature from around the world documents the use of a wide variety of inhalants among different ethnic and minority groups and the use of different types of inhalant from group to group. Young (1987) notes that in North America preferences for various inhalants differ according to ethnic groups, so that spray paints are preferred by Hispanics; correcting fluid and adhesive cements by Blacks;

and petrol, shoe polish and amyl nitrates by non-Hispanic whites. American Indian youth most commonly inhales petrol, followed by, in order of preference, glue or aerosol sprays (Young 1987). Indian groups using petrol as an inhalant include Pueblo (Kaufman 1973); Navaho (Coulehan et al 1983); and Plains Indians (Schottstaedt and Bjork 1977). Petrol sniffing is also practised by Mexican–American youth (Lund et al 1978; de la Fuente 1983) and by poor Brazilian youth in South America (Carlini-Cotrim and Carlini 1988). Benzine sniffing has been noted in the Pacific on Kiribati (Daniels and Fazakerley 1983) and among Black South African children (Moosa and Loening 1981). Petrol sniffing has commenced recently on Truk in Micronesia (M Marshall, personal communication) and has been practised for several years in New Zealand by Islanders and Maoris (Brown 1983).

STUDIES OF REGIONAL VARIATION OVERSEAS

Regional differences in the prevalence of petrol sniffing are occasionally remarked on, but rarely analysed. My study found notable regional variations in Australia, and I later offer some suggestions as to why this should be so. In terms of attempting to understand petrol sniffing (as one form of substance abuse) from the perspective of regional and cultural variation, studies from Canada offer some data. Among Canadian native peoples, sniffing is widespread in certain regions of the country, as it is in Australia. Manitoba is one Canadian province widely documented as having several communities where petrol sniffing is chronic (Stryde 1977; Seshia et al 1978; Boeckx et al 1977; Barnes 1980; Solvent Abuse Committee 1987), although north-west Ontario and northern Quebec are also mentioned (Smart et al 1986; Shkilnyk 1985). Little or no sniffing has been reported from the Yukon for twenty years, while, in the neighbouring Northwest Territories, sniffing is a continuing issue among native groups. Indigenous groups in Canada had (and still have in many regions) a similar socio-economic organisation (hunting, fishing and gathering) to Australian Aborigines. While the native involvement in the fur trade in Canada marks a significant historical and economic difference between indigenous people in Canada and in Australia, there are similarities between the effects of government policies in these countries. The other startling similarities between Australia and Canada can be found in the impact of government policies and white settlement on these indigenous forms of social organisation (Brody 1975).

Anthropological accounts of life in native Canadian villages have graphically documented the impact of white intrusion, and refer to the use of petrol as an inhalant by the youth of those communities (Brody 1975; Shkilnyk 1985). Both researchers interpret sniffing as a means of coping with day-to-day existence in isolated and stressed communities.

Brody wrote a detailed account of daily life in the Inuit villages of northern Canada which sets the scene for the desire to increase excitement (Brody 1975, 208–9):

> Time weighs heavily on the young. Those who feel unable or disinclined to hunt and trap must spend many hours trying to amuse themselves, by meandering here and there in the villages, visiting, gossiping, sitting, dreaming. In such a monotonous round, it is not surprising that they welcome the diversion of drink and the soft drugs that occasionally find their way even into the remotest settlements, and that they sometimes experiment with alcohol-substitutes, such as drinking after-shave lotion and sniffing gasoline. It is still rare to hear of excesses in such entertainment, but as settlement life develops these opportunities will increase. There is a growing interest in being intoxicated or high.

Shkilnyk worked much further south among Ojibwa Indians living in the lake and river systems of northwest Ontario. Her book proved to be controversial, in part because of her frank portrayal of social disorder (Shkilnyk 1985, 44–45):

> Perhaps the most insidious form of coping is the use of gasoline to get high. Sniffing gas is a form of escape from reality that is widely used, especially by the children of heavy drinkers. Like drinking for the adults, it is a social activity. Several children have already been severely burned by lighting cigarettes while sniffing, but the risk of immolation has not been a strong enough deterrent against this practice. The risk of physical burning of the body by accidental ignition of the gas has a parallel in the popular use of the word 'burnt' to describe the permanent destruction of brain cells by lead poisoning.
>
> The incidence of gas sniffing is not recorded in official documents for it is considered to be neither a crime nor a disease. Within the community, few seem to have noticed that so many children are slowly poisoning themselves. ... Of the twenty-four children in grade two in 1979, ten were sniffing heavily and showing signs of mental disorientation. Over half the children in grade three were sniffing gas. Grade four had a class of twenty children, six of them in an advanced state of intellectual and emotional derangement due to mixing gas with alcohol.

Shkilnyk paints a bleak and shocking picture of life at a village in the far west of Ontario, where incest, violence and suicide are common, along with petrol sniffing. She takes care to explain that this has come about 'when people are subjected to fundamental change, at a rate far beyond their ability to cope, in every single aspect of their culture simultaneously' (Shkilnyk 1985, 241). The basis for the disintegration of the community, according to Shkilnyk, lies primarily in its relocation from an old reserve adjoining a river (a main source of livelihood) to another site eight kilometres away. Other researchers, however, have pointed out that relocation has been a 'more or less universal event in the history of northern native communities' (Usher 1987, 42). Significantly, there is no evidence to suggest a consistent association between relocation and social disintegration in Canadian native communities; while some have never recovered (especially those moved long distances), others have suffered little. All have undergone rapid, forced social change. The alternative explanation, which Shkilnyk believes to be secondary, lies in the fact that the river became contaminated with mercury pollution from a paper mill, causing the loss of a local fishery, which was not just economically important to two native communities, but had also been a central social institution in the lives of the people.[1] This was a unique event that drastically affected the local communities, bringing a loss of direction and a sense of despair which manifested itself in social destruction and chronic substance abuse by adults and children alike.

The case is salutary as an example of the difficulties of finding what appear to be the underlying 'causes' of self-destructive substance abuse, and highlights the drawbacks associated with studies of a single community rather than comparisons between peoples experiencing similar social and political upheaval.[2]

Another social study conducted in Canada surveyed seven communities for petrol-sniffing activities and made an attempt to discover why some communities experienced the practice and not others, and why some were more dislocated than others (Stryde 1977). Stryde found that sniffing was practised in three out of seven communities by young people aged from six to eighteen years. Discussing the aetiology of the practice in each community, Stryde (1977, 57) comments,

> This is a question on which everyone has an opinion. Generally, these opinions cite one causative factor to the exclusion of all others. Poverty, lack of recreation, poor education, irresponsibility, parental alcoholism, cultural disintegration, acculturative stress, peer pressure, experimentation for kicks, stupidity and self-genocide have all been touted in their turn as the 'real reason' for gas sniffing. Perhaps the actual genesis of gas sniffing contains elements of all of these. Perhaps only some of these factors, plus others not identified, are involved. Perhaps

the actual causes vary with the community and with the individual. We do not know.³

Through his research, Stryde realised that not only may the causes of petrol sniffing be peculiar to the individual, but they may also be peculiar to each community. It is unlikely that potential causes are mutually exclusive, either in Canada or in Australia. Stryde found striking variations between communities, even between two separate communities who were once part of the same Indian band. In this instance the band split at some time in the past: one group (Shamattawa) now has a petrol-sniffing problem, the other (York Landing) does not. This often leads to conjecture over how two communities with the same recent roots could be so different in this one respect. The Shamattawa people were said to have 'an unenviable reputation for alcoholism, violence, gasoline sniffing and other social problems', with almost universal petrol sniffing among the children (Boeckx et al 1977, 142). On the other hand, despite an alcohol abuse problem, York Landing people discovered sniffing only occasionally and in all cases a meeting between the band chief, the parents and the child concerned had had positive results. Their main problem was watching out for visiting sniffers from Shamattawa, and extended visits of this kind were strongly discouraged by the chief and other community members. Both communities are isolated, and suffer from year-round unemployment and dependence on social security payments. The housing at York Landing was said to be poor, with no sewage treatment, and outdoor toilets. There were few social services and only one telephone. But York Landing did have strong leadership and a high level of concern for children's welfare. It is undoubtedly significant (as is the case in some Aboriginal communities) that immediate action was taken by community leaders, on a one-to-one basis, when sniffing was discovered.

Stryde (1977, 45) makes a useful suggestion in his concluding remarks, saying that

> It might be possible to understand when and by what means it [petrol sniffing] was introduced into each community. This is not simply a question of intellectual curiosity. Even a rough description of the genesis and dispersion paths of gasoline sniffing in Manitoba would be instructive in determining the conditions conducive to both.

Of course, this is no easy task as he discovered when attempting to document the social indicators associated with the presence or absence of sniffing. For example, one community with chronic sniffing was on reserved treaty land (ie holding secure title), and had a variety of sports and recreation facilities, including a community hall with dances and bingo. In communities with no sniffing he found strong leadership, clubs and organisations for almost every activity, and high levels of concern over children's welfare.

In contrast with the studies cited above, the medical and psychiatric literature barely touches upon such complex variables and confounding facts, and, when it does, it tends to reinforce bland generalisations. Remington and Hoffman (1984) assert that sniffing is more common in 'isolated' Indian reservations and they note that the community whose children they treated was experiencing high unemployment. Barnes (1985, 145) observes that the highest rates of sniffing were in the 'poorest' communities, while sniffing was absent in relatively rich ones. The data sources for these studies are clinical notes, sometimes self-report surveys, and quick background sketches of the home communities of hospital in-patients being treated for lead toxicity. Occasionally some data of sociological interest is included. Coulehan and colleagues (1983, 115), reporting on petrol-related morbidity among Navaho adolescents, noted that fifteen out of their twenty-three patients belonged to

> four separate groups, each composed of siblings and friends who sniffed gasoline together…Ten were judged to have inadequate parental supervision, nine had older siblings who sniffed gasoline, and parental alcohol abuse was recorded in four instances.

Because medical and psychiatric researchers often deal with samples of users, rather than looking at the wider population (or several groups), it is to be expected that such a selective group will reveal a variety of psycho-social problems. So it is that sniffers are said to come from broken homes and low socio-economic backgrounds, and are said to be insecure and have 'marginal intellectual capabilities' (see Cole et al 1986; Lund et al 1978). Researchers who look more widely into their populations have obtained different findings. Kaufman, for example, surveyed sniffers and non-sniffers in a Pueblo village school and found that the incidence of alcoholism was almost identical in the homes of both groups. The incidence of 'broken homes' did not differ greatly between the two groups either (Kaufman 1973). In their psychiatric study of Aboriginal petrol sniffers on Elcho Island in the Northern Territory, Nurcombe et al (1970) also found no significant differences in type of home, family prestige, presence or absence of parents, scholastic progress and command of English between sniffers and non-sniffers. Kaufman (1973, 1063) has an interesting suggestion to explain this disturbing 'normality':

> It is possible that as drug use becomes more prevalent in a community, it is increasingly accepted as normal behaviour.

Because of this acceptance, the population of users comes increasingly to resemble the population of abstainers in all other characteristics. A historical analogy with coffee drinkers and marijuana smokers is applicable.

A study of solvent users (including petrol sniffers) in Sao Paulo, Brazil, produced findings that were in accordance with those of Kaufman. Seventy-five per cent of sniffers lived with their own families and 16 per cent with one parent; 'almost the same percentage of non-users shared similar family situations' (Carlini-Cotrim and Carlini 1988). However, heavy alcohol use by one family member was found to be more common among solvent users in this study. The authors noted that although social minorities in Brazil constitute a high-risk population for solvent use, its use is increasing and 'spreading to other social levels'. It seemed to be a less stigmatised drug than others mentioned in their survey, as no-one refused to answer questions on solvent use. Although these researchers sampled 1,800 students from ten schools in four different areas of Sao Paulo, the one variable they did not investigate was regional/neighbourhood variation.

REGIONAL VARIATION IN AUSTRALIA

There are three regions in Australia where the use of petrol as an inhalant is endemic: parts of Arnhem Land, Northern Territory; Central Australia, in the regions intersected by the borders of South and Western Australia and the Northern Territory, and the far north of South Australia; and the Eastern Goldfields, including Kalgoorlie, Leonora and Laverton, in Western Australia. The use of petrol is reported in a few scattered Aboriginal communities apart from these three regions: five in Queensland; one in the Torres Strait, which appears to be anomalous; at least two in rural New South Wales; and three in rural South Australia. Table 2 provides an estimated distribution of affected communities according to data on the Department of Aboriginal Affairs (DAA) *Community Profiles* for 1985.

As this table shows, according to admittedly approximate estimations, fifty-six communities (6.7 per cent) out of a total of 837 throughout the country are said to have had petrol sniffing at the time of the data collection. From fieldwork and further investigation, it can be said that at least a few of the communities listed no longer have a problem, and several who do have incidences of petrol sniffing are not listed. Table 2 does not include the prevalence of petrol sniffing among urban populations, as the collection is confined to defined 'communities' (ie settlements, outstations, town camps and other groups). Nevertheless this estimation provides an overview of the prevalence of petrol sniffing in each state or territory. Of note is the fact that the two states with the largest proportion of the total Aboriginal population of Australia (Queensland and New South Wales) have very little reported petrol sniffing. On the other hand, South Australia, with only 6.28 per cent of the total Aboriginal population notes sixteen communities with petrol sniffing (including the six communities noted under the Northern Territory).

Apart from the DAA *Community Profiles*, the only other published source of data is the *Survey of Drug and Alcohol Use by Aboriginal School Students in New South Wales* in 1986 (NSW Aboriginal Education Consultative Group, 1986). As mentioned earlier, this survey asked students to nominate how many others they knew who used substances, and petrol was included on the list of solvents. The authors noted with concern that young people in certain regions were experimenting with 'dangerous combinations' of drugs (eg Coca-cola and petrol; wine and spirits, including methylated spirits). Inhalant use was more prevalent in some regions with 56 per cent of reports occurring in the western and Riverina regions of New South Wales. The use of petrol was more common in the Riverina, while glue sniffing was more common in the western region and the use of thinners

Table 2: Aboriginal communities reporting petrol sniffing in 1985 and Aborigines as a percentage of the population by state

State/Territory	Percentage of total Aboriginal population	No of communities	No of communities with sniffing
Queensland/TSI	26.91	81	4
New South Wales	25.92	84	2
Western Australia	16.6	165	11
Northern Territory	15.26	439	29*
South Australia	6.28	63	10
Victoria	5.54	2	nil
Tasmania	2.95	2	nil
Aust. Cap. Terr.	0.54	1	nil
Total	100%	837	56

* Six communities listed in DAA's Northern Territory profile are in fact in South Australia (Angatja, Aparawatatja, Kalka, Pipalyatjara, Pukatja and PutaPuta).

(Source: ABS and John Done, Statistics Section, Department of Aboriginal Affairs *Community Profiles*, 1985)

was noted in the metropolitan east. Of 110 reports of petrol sniffing, thirty-nine (35 per cent) came from the Riverina. The authors conclude:

> It is impossible for this study to determine the reasons for these regional differences. Possibly boredom is a greater factor in rural regions than it is in the city or maybe other forms of drugs and alcohol are more readily available in the city than they are in country areas. Whatever the reasons, however, it appears that there are definite regional differences and these should be taken into account when developing drug and alcohol education programs.

As the maps of the prevalence of sniffing in each state (Figures 1–5) show, some communities where sniffing has been reported in New South Wales

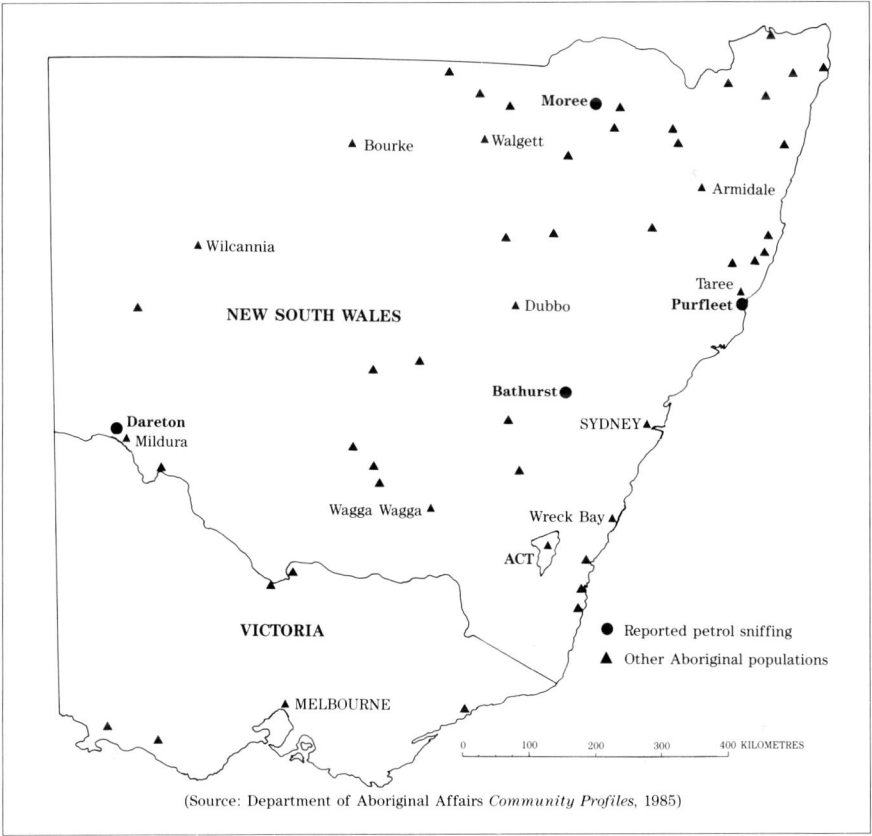

(Source: Department of Aboriginal Affairs *Community Profiles*, 1985)

Figure 1: The distribution of Aboriginal communities in New South Wales showing those that have reported petrol sniffing up to 1985

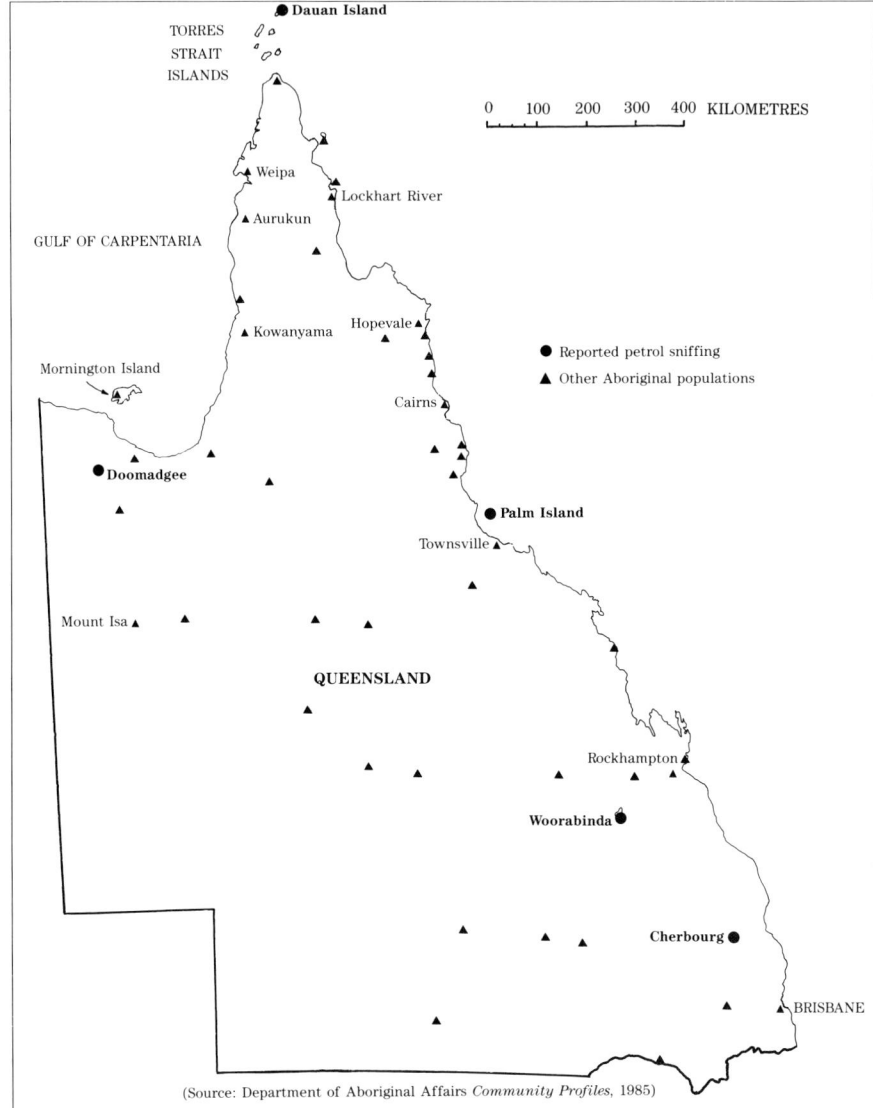

Figure 2: The distribution of Aboriginal communities in Queensland showing those that have reported petrol sniffing up to 1985

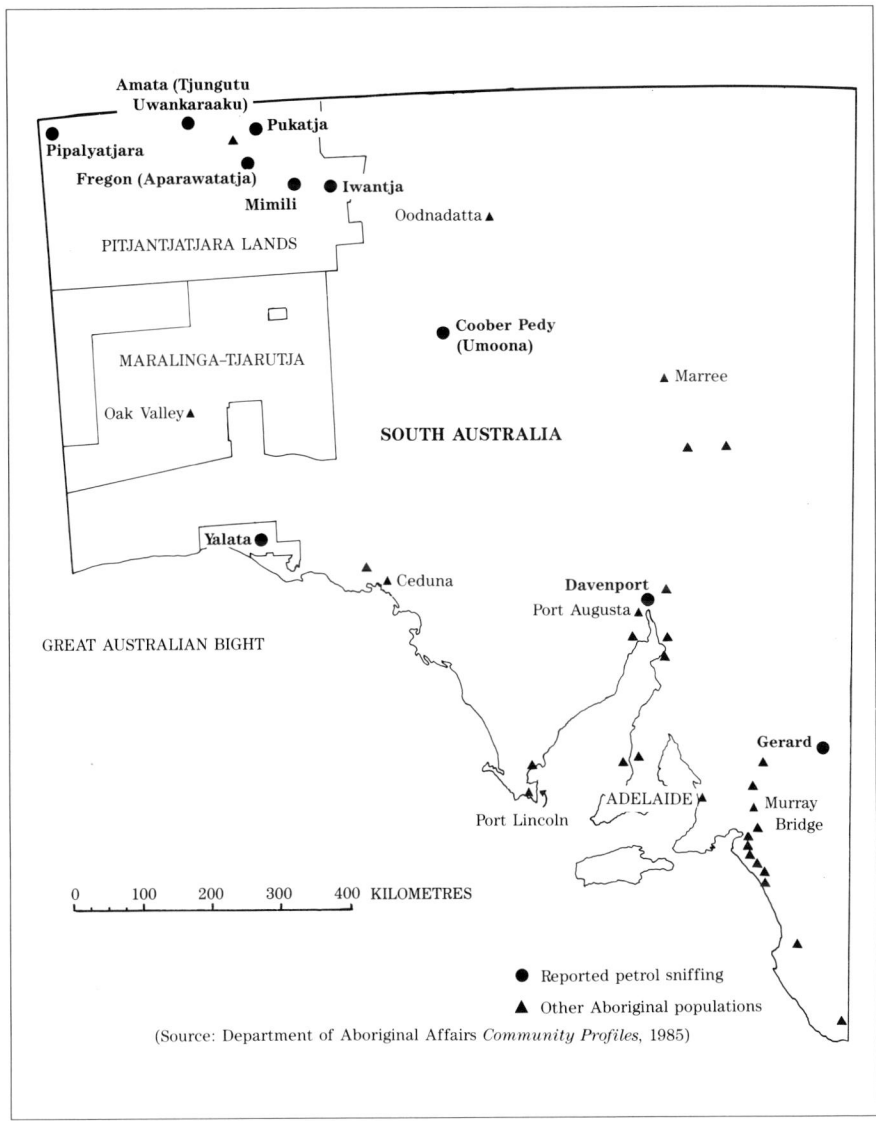

Figure 3: The distribution of Aboriginal communities in South Australia showing those that have reported petrol sniffing up to 1985

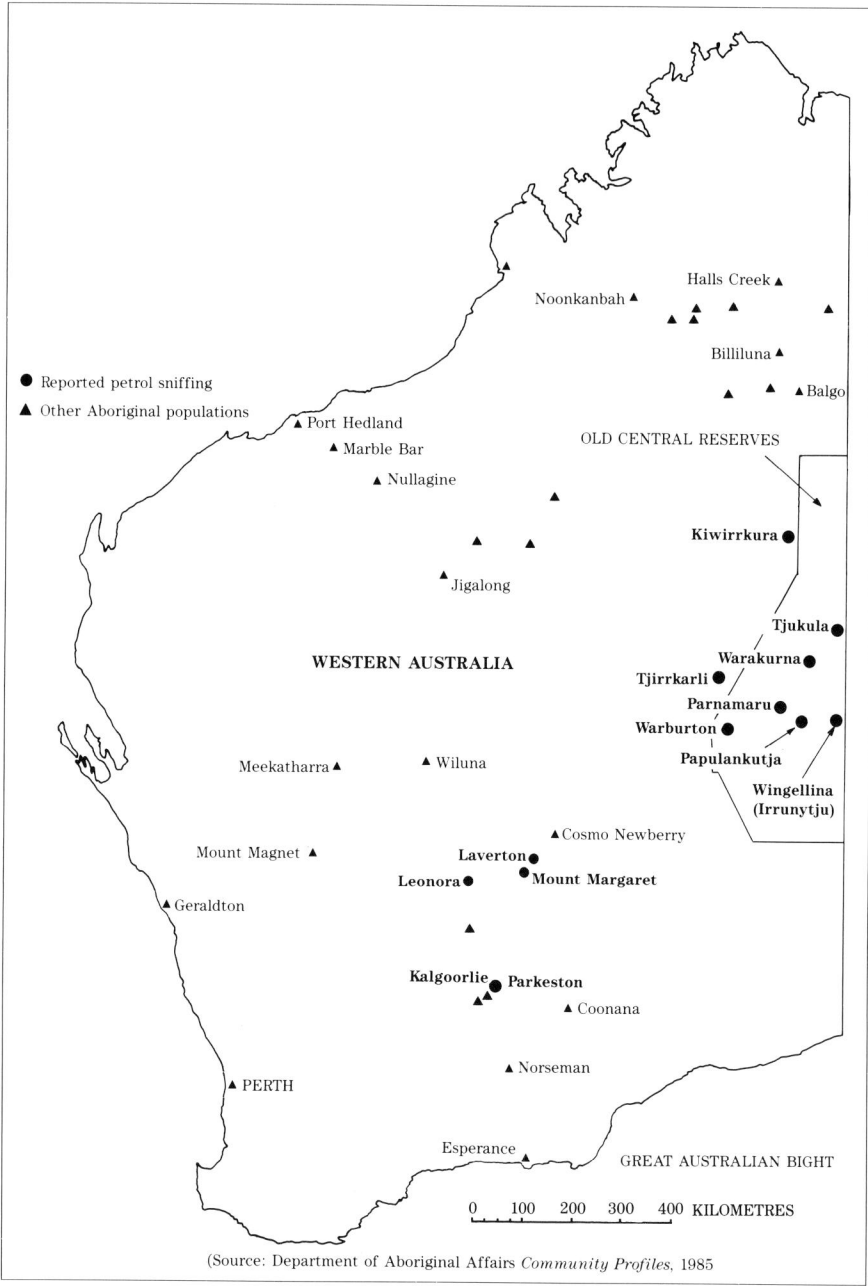

Figure 4: The distribution of Aboriginal communities in Western Australia showing those that have reported petrol sniffing up to 1985

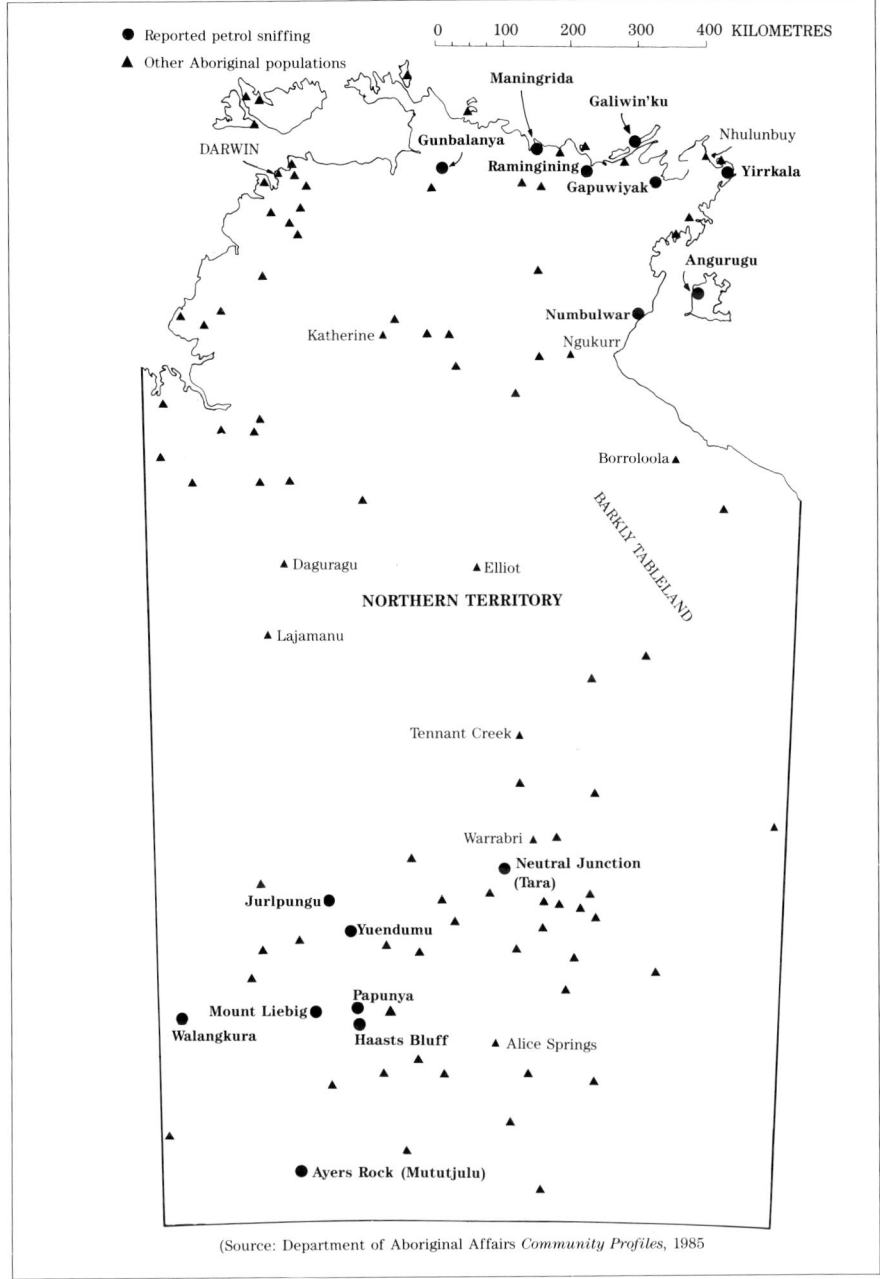

Figure 5: The distribution of Aboriginal communities in the Northern Territory showing those that have reported petrol sniffing up to 1985

and Queensland are geographically isolated from each other. In Western Australia, the Northern Territory and South Australia on the other hand, the petrol-using communities are, for the most part, geographically close. They are also socially and culturally close to one another. However, it is not a simple matter of closely associated communities becoming 'inoculated' by contact with sniffers,[4] as suggested by the Senate Select Committee (Commonwealth of Australia 1985, 163). A quick look at the maps will show that, although there are clusters of communities with endemic sniffing, others nearby (and others visited by sniffers) have not apparently been 'infected' (if we continue with the, perhaps unfortunate, analogy). The maps have been drawn to show the proximity of 'sniffing' communities (marked by a solid dot) to those not reported to have petrol sniffing (marked by a triangle). One notable anomaly is Aurukun in Queensland (Figure 2), which has no instances of petrol sniffing despite the existence of numerous other social problems, and despite its associations with Angurugu on Groote Eylandt through marriage links and church visits (Figure 5). Angurugu youths sniff petrol quite openly (Figure 5). Another anomaly is Borroloola, which has no petrol sniffing, despite close links with Numbulwar and Groote Eylandt (Figure 5) and Doomadgee in Queensland (Figure 2) which do have sniffing. Milingimbi (Figure 5), though having had an incidence of sniffing in the past (1950s–1960s), had a long period without the use of petrol that lasted until 1989. Milingimbi people interact frequently with those from Ramingining and Galiwin'ku, communities where sniffing occurs.

In Western Australia the communities clustered in the cld Central Reserves, where sniffing has been practised since the early 1970s, have ceremonial and other associations with Wiluna, where there is no sniffing (Figure 4). Petrol sniffing does not occur among residents of Jigalong, but its ceremonial links are primarily with other non-sniffing populations such as Wiluna, Nullagine and Marble Bar. Balgo is another population with links to non-sniffing communities to its north, but it has visitors from Kiwirrkurra and Yuendumu (NT), who occasionally engage in the practice.

While petrol sniffing is generally prevalent among populations who share linguistic, cultural and ceremonial associations (or a combination of all these), it is not inevitable that all such communities necessarily show an incidence of the practice. Some do not. However, it is possible to assert that populations whose primary associations are with other 'non-sniffing' populations rarely, if ever, have to deal with an incidence of petrol sniffing (eg Jigalong, Fitzroy Crossing, Halls Creek and Broome in Western Australia, and the Barkly Tableland populations in the Northern Territory). The vexed and anomalous question of the distribution of, and resistance to, the practice is taken up again shortly.

NOTES

1. I am grateful to Canadian anthropologist Jill Torrie, of the University of Toronto, for bringing this difference in interpretation to my attention.

2. The postscript to this case study is positive. A financial settlement was eventually agreed upon between all the parties; the native groups, the provincial and federal governments and the corporate polluters. A crisis intervention program started in the context of the financial settlement (Jill Torrie, personal communication). The program involved community members patrolling the community, taking petrol away from sniffers, taking people home, and preventing people doing 'foolish things' (Draper, 1985).

3. A similar list of 'real' causes of petrol sniffing in Australia may be found in the report of the Senate Select Committee on Volatile Substance Fumes (Commonwealth of Australia 1985, 163).

4. The committee utilised this term which, ironically, has two meanings: either to 'communicate a disease by inserting its aetiologic agent' or to 'introduce antigenic material for preventative, curative or experimental purposes' (Taylor 1988, 840). Heroin has been referred to as the 'junk virus' by one author (Kohn 1987, 144).

CHAPTER

3 SO TOXIC A SUBSTANCE

THE TOXICITY OF PETROL

In 1921, when United States research workers in the laboratories of General Motors discovered that organo-lead compounds acted as an antiknock agent in petrol, it was already known that these compounds were highly toxic. After thirteen deaths associated with the increased production of leaded petrol occurred, a public outcry in the United States in 1925 halted production for a year. Grandjean observed in 1983 that if the discovery had been made more recently, the addition to petrol of so toxic a substance would not be permitted (Grandjean 1983, 179, 186).

Despite the introduction of unleaded petrol in Australia in recent years, it will be a long time before unleaded vehicles are in common use by Aboriginal people in remote areas. Meanwhile, the use of leaded petrol as an inhalant by young Aboriginal people will continue to be associated with acute encephalopathy (degenerative disease of the brain), seizures, choreo-athetoid (involuntary jerky) movements and hallucinations — symptoms which require emergency trips to hospital. Children who survive acute encephalopathy are often left with permanent neurological sequelae and with mental impairment (Rutter 1980). Organo-lead compounds are readily absorbed through the respiratory and gastrointestinal tracts and the brain is the organ most sensitive to lead toxicity. Children inhaling petrol fumes absorb organic rather than inorganic lead. These organic lead compounds behave very differently from inorganic lead. Tenenbein and colleagues (1984, 1078) in Winnipeg, Manitoba, reported:

> Exposure to inorganic lead is well known to produce peripheral neuropathy. However, the lead in gasoline is organic. In the over 200 cases of intentional inhalation of leaded gasoline fumes evaluated at our hospital over the past decade...no case of clinical peripheral neuropathy had been documented.

So far, comparatively limited research attention has been paid to organic lead toxicity (Grandjean 1983, 185; Morice et al 1981). For this reason there is considerable uncertainty surrounding the diagnosis and treatment of symptoms associated with the sniffing of leaded petrol.

A full description of the acute and chronic effects of sniffing leaded petrol is provided in Morice et al (1981) and in a Commonwealth Department of Health Information Paper (1985). In short, the initial effects of acute exposure may include the following, listed by Grandjean (1983): anorexia, vomiting, insomnia, tremor, weakness, fatigue, headache, aggression, depression, irritability, body pains, restlessness, hyperactivity, difficulties in concentrating, confusion, impairment of memory and strange sensations. All these symptoms will be familiar to Aboriginal health workers and community health nurses in settlements where petrol sniffing is prevalent. Anorexia and subsequent weight loss among petrol sniffers is frequently reported in the medical literature (Keenlyside 1984; Grandjean 1984; Brown 1983; Carroll and Abel 1973; Eastwell 1979; Freeman 1985; Wardaguga and Dawumal 1980). Experimental studies of rats injected with leaded and unleaded petrol found that both groups lost weight, with the leaded petrol group being more seriously affected (Saito 1973). Following the acute reactions, Grandjean (1983, 183) observed that hours or even days may pass before

> a serious exacerbation occurs in the form of acute mania, convulsions, delirium, fever and coma... . In serious cases, death has followed in 36 hours or after several days. The longer the period until symptoms set in or become aggravated, the better the prognosis.

LEAD ABSORPTION

The published literature on lead absorption pertains to the effects of inorganic rather than organic lead. This makes estimation of the amount of lead inhaled by petrol sniffers extremely difficult. The following brief discussion thus refers only to inorganic lead, with consequent uncertainty as to its applicability to sniffers (Milton Tenenbein, personal communication). Young children are most susceptible to lead toxicity: the maximum uptake of lead occurs during the second and third year of life (McMichael et al 1988, 470). However, there is a high individual variability in lead absorption among children (Mahaffey 1982, 65). Luckily most children who use petrol are somewhat older than this, although neuropathy is reported from overseas in a four-year-old Sudanese boy who sniffed petrol (Hall et al 1986, 900–1), and there are anecdotal reports of very young Aboriginal children inhaling petrol fumes. It appears that the brain generally becomes less sensitive to external influences with increasing age (Medical Research Council 1983, 4). High inorganic lead levels among very young children are usually associated with pica (the eating of non-food substances such as paint), although the studies associated with the lead smelters at Port Pirie, South Australia, involve a cohort of 537 children born between 1979 and 1982 exposed to environmental lead (McMichael et al 1988). It is not known at what age children's absorption of lead changes to adult patterns (Mahaffey 1982, 66), but young people categorised by Glass (1981) as 'children' were said to absorb up to 40 per cent of ingested (not inhaled) lead. In adults, the usual level of absorption (in a non-fasting state) is said to be between 5 and 10 per cent, again with individual variations (Mahaffey 1982, 65).[1] The lethal dose to humans of tetraethyl lead (the toxic lead added to petrol) is approximately one quarter of a gram (Grandjean 1983, 186).

HYDROCARBON TOXICITY

Apart from tetraethyl lead, or more rarely tetramethyl lead, petrol contains other potential toxins. Kaelen et al (1986,806) list these as the aromatic hydrocarbons such as benzene, toluene, xylene and the naphthalenes, paraffins and alkenes. In its submission to the Senate Select Committee on Volatile Substance Fumes, the Commonwealth Department of Health prepared a detailed analysis of the composition and toxicity of volatile hydrocarbons (Senate Select Committee 1985, 5-120). The amounts of hydrocarbons in petrol are unpredictable, and so it is difficult to generalise about their potential toxicities (Press and Done 1967). Significantly, Seshia and colleagues observe that the neurological manifestations of petrol sniffing could be caused by any one, or all, of the constituents in petrol, and/or hydrocarbons (Seshia et al 1978; Grandjean 1983, 180).

Coulehan et al (1983) discuss the relative contributions to morbidity of tetraethyl lead and hydrocarbons in petrol. Their study examined petrol sniffing among Navaho adolescents, and they divided symptomatic cases into two groups: those with acute toxic encephalopathy (nineteen in number), and those with subacute neurologic symptoms such as tremor and ataxia (numbering fourteen). Both syndromes are consistent with reported cases of apparent tetraethyl lead toxicity. In an attempt to discover whether the syndromes they observed were caused by lead or by the hydrocarbons, the researchers examined the evidence for adverse effects. Coulehan et al note that petrol contains a volatile component, N-Hexane, which can cause polyneuropathy (disease of parts of the nervous system), a condition clinically similar to inorganic lead poisoning, but none of their patients showed polyneuropathy. They conclude that the bulk of evidence suggests that tetraethyl lead toxicity is paramount in these patients, but they would not rule out the possibility that aliphatic (fatty) hydrocarbons contribute to the acute delirium and excitement (Coulehan et al 1983, 116). It is often supposed that the removal of lead from petrol will eventually reduce the morbidity associated with petrol sniffing, but the Institute of Petroleum, in its submission to the Senate Select Committee, points out that 'the contrary may be true, since one effect of removing the lead from petrol is that the concentration of aromatic hydrocarbons increases' (Commonwealth of Australia 1985, 189). Unleaded petrol has a higher hydrocarbon (benzine) content than the ordinary product (and so is potentially more dangerous) but, according to a spokesperson for the Australian Institute of Petroleum, it does not contain the heavy metal manganese, as was suggested to the Senate Select Committee (Commonwealth of Australia, Sydney Hearings 1985, 728; R Corinaldi, Australian Institute of Petroleum, personal communication).

The syndrome of 'sudden sniffing death' is associated with the volatile hydrocarbons in petrol, rather than with organolead compounds such as tetraethyl lead. Vaporisation occurs more rapidly in hot weather. Bass (1970) documents five cases of sudden sniffing death, three of which were associated with siphoning petrol in hot weather. He concludes (1970, 203):

> Stress or vigorous activity after sniffing abuse of gasoline mixtures or other volatile hydrocarbons is associated with the sudden-death event. The mechanism of sudden death is the result of a hydrocarbon induced spontaneous cardiac arrythmia.

Hydrocarbons, then, are perhaps more significant than is commonly thought. While lead is undoubtedly a highly toxic component in petrol, it would be a mistake to underestimate the contribution of the toxic volatile hydrocarbons to the symptoms that chronic petrol sniffers experience.

ENCEPHALOPATHY

There are several key published accounts which document cases of inhalation-induced encephalopathy. These include a report on two Canadian Indian youths by Boeckx et al (1977); accounts of chelation treatment (used in the treatment of heavy metal poisoning) and deaths in native Americans (Valpey et al 1978; Coulehan et al 1983); a case report from New Zealand (Brown 1983); and two separate reports of encephalopathy in Australian Aboriginal patients (Kaelen et al 1986; Rischbieth et al 1987).

These reported cases reveal that there is considerable variation in individual responses to elevated blood lead levels and to treatment. Lengths of stay in hospital vary considerably, both in published research accounts and in the Aboriginal community health records I perused. Several young petrol sniffers who were hospitalised from Arnhem Land communities stayed in the Royal Darwin Hospital for only eight days while receiving chelation therapy. In Western Australia the length of stay has decreased from an average of 20.2 days in 1981 to 7.86 in 1986 for all cases where petrol sniffing was noted as the 'principal' or 'other' condition contributing to hospital stay (Hayward and Kickett 1988, 17). Experienced Canadian physicians treating solvent abusers generally recommend that the detoxification period in chronic abusers should be as long as possible: 'at least two weeks of close observation are necessary for the brain of these young

Table 3: Hospital treatment and outcome in eight cases of petrol-related encephalopathy

Authors	Location	Length of stay	Treatment	Outcome
Boeckx et al (1977) (two cases)	Winnipeg, Canada	(1) 4 weeks (2) 10 weeks (3) 72 hours	EDTA, BAL, Penacillamine Penacillamine dilantin	readmitted later readmitted later death
Valpey et al (1978)	Seattle, USA	(1) 3 weeks (2) 6 weeks (3) 17 days	EDTA, BAL Penacillamine no treatment	readmitted later readmitted later discharged 'normal'
		(1) 5 days? (2) 4 weeks (3) 4 weeks (4) 3 days	Penacillamine EDTA, BAL, Penacillamine EDTA, BAL none	readmitted readmitted readmitted death
Brown (1983)	Hamilton, New Zealand	(1) 26 days	EDTA, BAL, Penacillamine	discharged, intellect dull
Kaelen et al (1986)	Perth, Western Australia	(1) 4 days	Dilantin	death
Rischbieth et al (1987) (two cases)	Adelaide, South Australia	(1) 6 weeks (1) 19 days	BAL, EDTA, Penacillamine BAL, EDTA	discharged, only mild improvement discharged, recovery
McGrath (1986)	Woolangabba, Queensland	(1) 4 weeks?	Chelation (no further details)	discharged, no significant residual deficits

EDTA = Calcium disodium edetate
BAL = British Anti-Lewisite

persons to be rid of the effect of the solvent' (Fornazzari 1988, 109). Table 3 shows length of stay, treatment and outcome for some published cases of petrol-related encephalopathy.

The following anonymous case histories of Australian Aboriginal patients from various regions provide some insight into the symptoms which must, in the first instance, be dealt with at the local clinic level. The data are derived from clinic records, interviews with Aboriginal health workers and sisters, my own field notes and coroners' records.

MB: a female from east Arnhem Land, born in 1961 (age twenty-six)
> This young woman was said to have sniffed 'twenty-four hours a day' (over an unspecified period). She suffered from sleeplessness and bizarre behaviour, and swam far out to sea on one occasion. She was treated locally with the tranquillisers Valium and Chlorpromazine, then evacuated to hospital in Darwin where she received chelation therapy.

NL: a male from east Arnhem Land, born in 1961 (age twenty-six)
> One of the first in his community to sniff petrol in 1980, this young man engaged in self-wounding behaviour, 'talking funny things' and occasionally fell off roofs. He was evacuated to Gove Hospital and treated with tranquillisers and has now ceased sniffing.

WP: a male from east Arnhem Land, born in 1961 (age twenty-six)
> Family members brought this young man to his community clinic suffering from strange behaviour and tremor; he was unable to walk straight or stand on one leg. He denied that there was anything wrong with him. He was treated with Valium and Chlorpromazine but did not respond to sedation and was evacuated to Darwin and chelated.

BR: a male from Western Australia, born in 1972 (age sixteen)
> This boy had inhaled petrol over a period of approximately ten years. Presenting variously with self-inflicted wounds, pneumonia, bizarre behaviour and once with a 'moving head', by 1986 he had a blood lead level of 111 micrograms of lead per decilitre of blood. His elderly parents had come to the clinic for help; the Department of Community Welfare had discussed and then dropped the case. After one unsuccessful attempt at evacuation, he was finally airlifted to a regional hospital where he died of pneumonia and lead poisoning. He was sixteen years old and weighed thirty kilograms.

LA: a male from Western Australia, born in 1968 (age twenty)
> At one year of age this boy was seen by clinic staff with malnutrition and anaemia. In 1985 (aged seventeen) he was thought to be a petrol

sniffer. Two weeks before his death in 1988 he presented with a sore throat, vomiting and lethargy. He was found on his bed in the early morning with no pulse or respiration and did not respond to resuscitation attempts. The cause of death was pulmonary congestion and pneumonia.

SN: a male from Western Australia, born in 1968 (age twenty-one)
This youth had presented four times in 1987 with fits and withdrawals from petrol sniffing. Two years later, weighing forty kilograms, he died in a city hospital after two weeks of treatment and resuscitation.

JT: a male from central Arnhem Land, born in 1967 (age twenty-one)
In 1986 and 1987 this young man was evacuated with symptoms associated with petrol sniffing. Fifteen months later his father reported the boy had twice had fits. The next day he presented at the clinic with tremor, having sniffed petrol all night. Three days later he twice had fits, despite treatment with Valium, and was evacuated to hospital suffering from agitation, disorientation and hallucinations, after having been unconscious in the community clinic throughout the day. After approximately six weeks in hospital and chelation therapy, he was discharged to attend a residential care program.

SH: a male from South Australia, born in 1964 (age twenty)
It was noted in 1978 that this boy sniffed petrol. His father had died the previous year from an alcohol-related fit. He was fined for illegal use of a motor car, and then in 1978 incarcerated in a juvenile detention centre for another illegal use. There he experienced what staff interpreted as withdrawal symptoms which took the form of cramps and visual hallucinations. He reportedly resolved to stop petrol sniffing. A social worker observed that he disliked the vomiting and dizziness which often comes directly after the fumes are inhaled, before the euphoria. After two months he was back in his community, where he fired a rifle three times at another adolescent. He was subsequently held on remand, but on the day he returned to the community he stole some petrol. Two months later his mother died from alcohol-related renal disease. He was fostered out to several different families and issued with a rations order from the welfare department to enable him to buy food and clothing. In January 1979, a local Department of Community Welfare officer described him in a report as being

erratic...sudden bursts of activity...laughing uncontrollably at small incidents. Relations say that he does silly things and talks in a silly way sometimes. There may be some degree of brain damage from petrol sniffing.

A blood lead test in 1979 showed that he had an elevated lead level. By the end of 1979, aged fifteen, he had appeared eighteen times in the Children's Court. In 1980 he was sent to another community where for a while he 'settled down and was sent to school'. In 1981 he returned to his home community and was thought by many community residents to be responsible for a rapid increase in petrol sniffing. He was frequently seen with a twelve-year-old boy, also a chronic sniffer. While community members blamed him for the upsurge in sniffing, he told social workers that he was angry at the amount of drinking at the community and said that his people had 'let him down'. In June 1981 he appeared in court again for an attempted sexual assault and larceny committed in a neighbouring town. In court the magistrate asked if the elders of the community would initiate him, in which case he would suspend the five-month sentence. After considering the matter, the men refused to incorporate the boy ritually on the grounds that he was 'too young'. He was therefore incarcerated in a juvenile institution. In 1984 he died at the age of twenty as a result of cardiac failure due to the inhalation of petrol fumes. A milk tin and a golden syrup tin, both containing a small amount of petrol, were found in the shed where he died (Ahern 1987; Brady and Morice 1982, 82–86).

RECOVERY

Recovery from the severe symptoms of chronic petrol sniffing is extremely variable and impossible to predict (Milton Tenenbein, personal communication). Varying degrees of recovery from lead toxicity are described in the published literature, but the prognosis is much more difficult to follow up in Australian Aboriginal cases. This is because patients often leave hospital to be admitted to 'rehabilitation' or residential programs, and also because distance and high population mobility can make it difficult to keep track of patients. City hospitals make no attempt to follow up their Aboriginal patients once they return to their communities. Additionally, community clinics often do not receive copies of all the documentation concerning their patients' stay in hospital; they do not always receive copies of coroners' reports if a death occurs. This makes ongoing monitoring of an ex-patient a challenging, though not insurmountable, problem.

Some of the published research provides useful data on recovery. Hall et al (1986) noted that their four-year-old sniffer (who was not chelated) showed minimal weakness and was able to walk seven months after suffering acute neuropathy. Brown (1983) reported that fifteen weeks after treatment with chelating agents a patient seemed normal, with a normal gait, but appeared intellectually dull. Seshia et al (1978) provide a detailed assessment of neurological manifestations at the fifth and the eighth weeks of monitoring. Only one patient (out of forty-six) had residual neurological signs at follow-up, but the authors caution that no psychological studies were done and so the level of mental 'retardation', if any, was not known. Boeckx et al (1977) noted that four weeks after admission and D-Penacillamine chelation treatment, the patient was still uncoordinated and tremulous; two months later he was 'normal'. Valpey et al (1978), however, report a progressive encephalopathy and they stress that, although earlier studies had thought encephalopathy to be reversible, the permanent changes in health and the later death of their patient were attributed to 'severe and repeated lead poisoning, as suggested by serum, urine and postmortem brain lead levels' (Valpey et al 1978, 509). Nevertheless, they conclude that if death can be averted during the acute phase then complete recovery appears to be the rule. Similarly, Grandjean (1984) observes that if a patient shows symptomatic improvement within three weeks, then he or she may survive. He stresses that a short latency period (between exposure and the onset of symptoms) suggests a grave prognosis.

    A review of the convalescence and recovery period after a serious intoxication with tetraethyl lead revealed that recovery may take from a few weeks to two years (Grandjean 1984, 233). At Maningrida, in the Northern Territory, despite the fact that twenty-five individuals have been hospitalised on one or more occasions from 1984 to 1988, and many more (up to sixty) are regular users of petrol, only two individuals show obvious ongoing neurological signs (Dr C Connors, personal communication). However, the non-specific nature of symptoms makes it very difficult to assess deficiencies such as intellectual impairment or decreased ability to learn, even in those users who appear to have recovered in other respects. Grandjean states unequivocally that the brain has only a limited potential to recover and that neuronal death cannot be repaired (Grandjean 1984, 236).

    Because of the difficulties of follow-up in Australia mentioned earlier, it is hard to estimate the recovery level among acutely intoxicated Aboriginal petrol sniffers. Certainly some sniffers regain their former physical coordination, and Aboriginal community members see them as 'cured'. However, community health staff can usually identify ex-sniffers, whom they describe as being 'slow', 'vegetable-like', 'happy but ga-ga' and 'uncontrollable and brain-damaged', suggesting that they have suffered some brain damage. One young woman of twenty, who was hospitalised and chelated on four occasions and who returned to her Arnhem Land community walking with the aid of a frame, often falls over and remains virtually silent more than one year after her last hospital stay.

CLINIC AND HOSPITAL TREATMENT

The most common way a toxic sniffer comes to the attention of community health staff in clinics is when a relative reports that a sniffer is having fits or behaving strangely, or when he or she brings the patient to the clinic. Sometimes the sniffer is unconscious. The most common treatment at this stage is sedation, usually with Diazepam (oral Valium), and sometimes with the more heavy duty Chlorpromazine. Fits are treated with intravenous Valium or Phenytoin (Dilantin, an anti-convulsant). Aboriginal parents sometimes perceive these treatments to be a 'cure' and bring their sniffers to clinics asking for a 'needle to quieten him down'. Morice et al (1981) provide acute treatment guidelines. Grandjean warns that drugs with a cortical effect, such as a morphine, are contra-indicated as a symptomatic treatment, as they can worsen the condition (Grandjean 1984, 236).

The decision to hospitalise or not, which in many Aboriginal communities in the bush involves aerial evacuation, rests largely with the local community health sister. Sisters in some regions can find making this decision, and implementing it, problematic. There are several reasons for these difficulties. First, because of high staff turnover, sisters alone in remote clinics may be temporary or agency nurses with no experience in the management of petrol inhalers. Second, if their health service does not employ its own medical practitioners, they may have difficulty obtaining the often sought advice of a doctor. For example, sisters working in the old Central Reserves region of Western Australia must radio to the Royal Flying Doctor Service (RFDS) base and consult a doctor there. There can be disagreement over the correct course of action, but the sisters usually have more first-hand experience with the acute symptoms of leaded petrol intoxication. Third, aerial evacuation may be difficult to arrange or may be delayed. In the Warburton region, for example, clinic sisters use the RFDS based in Kalgoorlie for evacuation, which involves usually more than the one and a half hours minimum direct flying time. A plane might have to make a special trip for such an evacuation, and aircraft must serve a large area of the Eastern Goldfields and Central Australia (Western Australia). The RFDS has indicated a general unwillingness to evacuate petrol sniffers from this region. If the RFDS plane is already out on call, it may be five hours before it can reach the community concerned. A night landing requires the airstrip to be lit, and sometimes this means that several vehicles have to be rounded up to illuminate the strip with their headlights.

Fourth, a sniffer has to be heavily sedated before he or she can be evacuated by air. Most aerial medical services class petrol-sniffing patients as 'psychiatric' cases, and will not carry them unless they are heavily sedated. Some patients are also restrained in straitjackets for evacuation. Fifth, there are as yet no formal procedures for health sisters to follow regarding evacuation of sniffers. They must rely on their own ability to detect the symptoms and neurological 'signs' indicating that a sniffer is suffering from chronic intoxication, rather than simply experiencing the acute effects of being 'high' on petrol. A fit, for example, can be a difficult symptom for sisters to interpret. Petrol sniffers often have seizures, but so do many other Aboriginal patients. Aboriginal usage of the term 'fit' or the phrase 'taking a fit' is very broad. Someone who coughs a lot, or gasps and splutters for air can be said to be 'taking a fit'. A drinker who temporarily becomes unconscious will be described as having had a 'fit'. Among Ngaanyatjarra community members (Western Australia), a fit may be interpreted as the outcome of a spirit entering a person through the soles of their feet, so that relatives of a petrol sniffer who is taken ill may ask that his feet be bandaged.

Another aspect to these perceptions of what constitutes a fit is that a fit evokes expressions of concern and compassion from others (epitomised in Pitjantjatjara, for example, in the word *ngaltutjara* 'poor thing'). A petrol sniffer who has been the recipient of hostility on the part of others may be suddenly treated with sympathy if he or she has a fit. Nursing sisters in several regions observe that some individuals bring on their own fits as attention-seeking behaviour, to the extent that a sister will give a placebo injection as treatment. A 'real' fit is indicated by incontinence and post-seizure grogginess among other signs. In short, if a nursing sister is called out to someone who is said to have had a fit, she or he cannot always be sure that a true seizure has occurred. Aboriginal people have their own treatments for fits: I saw Warburton people treating an alcohol-related fit by stroking the patient's palms and fingers and calling out 'Wake up! Wake up!'.

CHELATION THERAPY IN AUSTRALIA

Chelating agents are chemical compounds which bind heavy metals, including lead. The derivation of the term is from the Greek *chele* meaning 'claw'. The use of chelating agents, however, assumes that tetraethyl lead is the chief toxic agent in leaded petrol. Some of the research findings presented in this chapter, together with the comments from Canadian toxicologists, suggest that this is not necessarily the case, and that hydrocarbons are at least equally responsible for the intoxication and symptomatology of petrol sniffers. Chelating agents may be given with intravenous or intramuscular injections, or taken orally. Probably as the result of the published work of Boeckx et al from Manitoba (1977), who were the first to evacuate native gasoline sniffers and treat them in hospital with chelating agents, intoxicated Aboriginal patients have been (and still are) chelated in Australia. The use of this treatment is not universal across Australia, however, as hospital physicians in different states and the Northern Territory disagree as to the efficacy and safety of the treatment. In Morice et al (1981, 29–33), a review of treatments with chelating agents is provided, including regimes for each agent. The three main chelating agents are briefly described below.

Calcium disodium edetate (EDTA) may be given with intramuscular injections, which are extremely painful even with a local anaesthetic. It can also be administered intravenously, in an infusion drip, which is less painful. This treatment may actually raise the lead level in an individual who is on the verge of encephalopathy, so British Anti-Lewisite (BAL) is used in conjunction with EDTA to counteract this effect. D-Penacillamine is another chelating agent, administered either by intramuscular injection or orally, the latter being used frequently in out-patient treatment. All these drugs cause lead to be excreted in the patient's urine. Sniffers treated with EDTA and BAL in city hospitals are often treated subsequently as out-patients in their home community, where the local clinic administers a course of oral Penacillamine. Continuing Penacillamine treatment is also conducted in gaol (in the Northern Territory) if an individual has been referred from gaol to hospital and then returns to complete a period of imprisonment.

Royal Darwin Hospital in the Northern Territory uses chelating agents for the treatment of petrol sniffers more frequently than any other hospital in Australia, with some individuals receiving chelation therapy on numerous occasions. All patients with signs of encephalopathy are sent to Darwin rather than Gove Hospital in east Arnhem Land, which is smaller and has no intensive care unit. In Darwin, the decision to chelate a patient is taken according to the clinical history provided by the patient's home clinic and the clinical assessment made at the hospital. Blood lead levels are usually unavailable for the assessment as the blood samples are sent to Brisbane.[2] Once a patient is in hospital, twenty-four-hour urinary lead and twice-weekly serum lead levels are taken. The hospital protocol for chelating a petrol sniffer with tetraethyl lead poisoning recommends a combined course of EDTA and BAL, with intravenous Valium for spasms and tremor. Patients are then started on low dose oral Penacillamine which is continued for two months once the patient is discharged.

Alice Springs Hospital in the Northern Territory has a policy of only using chelating agents for those with 'severe symptoms and elevated blood lead levels'. In the last quarter of 1986 there was an 'epidemic' of intoxication among petrol sniffers, in which approximately seventy-five patients were admitted to the hospital. According to Dr MG Kirubakaran, Specialist Physician at Alice Springs Hospital (personal communication),

> The severity of intoxication varied widely and patients with mild or moderate symptoms were treated conservatively. Chelating agents were used only for the severe cases with symptoms of encephalopathy.... . Apparently the response to chelating agents was good in most patients, but the very severe cases ended up with residual neurological deficits of varying degrees.

Alice Springs Hospital has a protocol for the management of petrol sniffing patients (1986) which includes:

1. intravenous fluids to maintain hydration;
2. sedation (Paraldehyde);
3. anti-epileptic medication (Phenytoin);
4. chelation therapy (Dimercaprol (BAL) 24 milligrams per kilogram of body weight per day intramuscularly in six doses for five days, EDTA 50 milligrams per kilogram of body weight per day intramuscularly in six doses for five days);
5. nutrition (nasogastric feeding or parenteral nutrition, ie feeding through the nose, by injection or intravenously).

The management protocol continues (Alice Springs Hospital 1986):

> Intensive nursing care is very important in the children's management. The children are normally nursed on a mattress on the floor. Constant attention is required to prevent self-inflicted injury when they thrash about and to care for IV fluids, nutrition, bowels and bladder.... . The agitation and myoclonic jerks [shocklike muscle contractions] often worsen after several days in hospital. The conscious state often remains depressed during chelation therapy. Following completion of chelation therapy, the sicker children have marked cerebellar inco-ordination and are unable to walk. Physiotherapy with the use of a walking frame or 4-pronged stick is useful at this stage.

In South Australia, the Adelaide Children's Hospital has chelated at least two Aboriginal petrol sniffers (Rischbieth et al 1987) and another individual (non-Aboriginal) who ingested contaminated water. A small number of children with raised blood lead levels associated with the Port Pirie lead smelter have been sent to Adelaide for chelation (Dr E Robertson, personal communication; McMichael et al 1988).

Western Australian hospitals, including Perth hospitals and Kalgoorlie Hospital, have so far used chelating agents extremely rarely, perhaps only in one or two cases. Kalgoorlie Hospital, the most usual reception point for intoxicated sniffers from the interior, is a 120-bed facility with two full-time doctors and an intensive care unit, but it has no formal program of detoxification. There have been reported problems in the management of petrol sniffers, as patients sometimes abscond into the town of Kalgoorlie. The hospital attempts to 'dry out' sniffers without resorting to the use of chelating agents, however, patients with multi-system failure must be sent to Perth hospitals. One case of encephalopathy resulting from petrol inhalation is reported from Queensland, in which a fifteen-year-old male was treated with EDTA and Penacillamine at Princess Alexandra Hospital, Woolangabba (McGrath 1986, 221). McGrath asserts that chelation therapy is 'today a safe and effective method of treatment'.

The overseas use of chelating agents for petrol sniffers appears to be widespread. Chelating agents have been used in the treatment of petrol-intoxicated sniffers in Winnipeg, Canada; Pittsburgh and Seattle, United States; and in New Zealand. Coulehan et al (1983) from Pittsburgh support the use of chelating agents on the grounds that chelation markedly increases the excretion of lead. They write: 'The statement that "chelating agents are of doubtful value" appears to be incorrect' (Coulehan et al 1983, 116).

This brief survey of treatment methods in Australia and overseas reveals some uncertainty over the efficacy of chelating agents in the treatment of petrol sniffers — an uncertainty which echoes a dispute among medical scientists over the use of these agents. Physicians in Winnipeg no longer chelate patients who have been abusing petrol unless it is absolutely necessary. The *United States Center for Disease Control Guidelines for Preventing Lead Poisoning in Young Children* (United States Department of Health, Education and Welfare 1978, 5) unequivocally states: 'intoxication due to tetraethyl lead and tetramethyl lead presents a special problem...chelating agents are not used'. Briefly, the causes for concern nominated by researchers are as follows:

1. Although reports in the 1960s and 1970s showed that chelating agents produced good results in the treatment of inorganic lead poisoning, there has always been doubt as to their effectiveness with organic lead poisoning, the type of poisoning experienced by petrol sniffers (Morice et al 1981, 33).

2. The risk of side effects from chelation therapy is not small. According to Dr E Robertson, Director of Chemical Pathology at Adelaide Children's Hospital (personal communication), Penacillamine, for example, may precipitate an acute reaction associated with kidney damage. 'Calcium EDTA may also produce kidney damage and BAL may produce liver damage' (Milton Tenenbein, personal communication).

3. The risk of kidney damage is increased if an individual is chelated more than once (Dr E Robertson, personal communication).

4. If exposure to lead continues while an individual is being treated with Penacillamine, the absorption of lead is actually increased (Dr E Robertson, personal communication).

5. Of most concern is a publication by Chisholm (1987)[3] who is considered to be a pioneer in the area of chelation therapy and the use of modern methods for the diagnosis and treatment of lead poisoning. His article suggests that the use of chelating agents is questionable, even in cases of inorganic lead poisoning where it was previously thought to be effective.

The basis of Chisholm's concern, expressed as 'a reappraisal' of the use of EDTA, is associated with what happens to the lead that has been mobilised. He presents data from animal studies which make it clear 'that synthetic metal-binding agents do have the potential to redistribute metals within the body' (Chisholm 1987, 1256). He cites a study (still in press at the time of his writing) which showed that treatment of rats with EDTA decreased blood, bone and renal lead levels 'but the brain level increased by up to 100 per cent over control values .... These data certainly raise concerns about the safety of the calcium disodium edetate mobilisation test, even in asymptomatic children with moderately increased lead absorption.' His concern was, in the first instance, over the use of the diagnostic EDTA mobilisation test — a test which has been proposed for use whenever chelation therapy is contemplated in children with blood lead levels in the range 1.21 to 2.65 micromols of lead per litre of blood (25 to 55 micrograms of lead per decilitre of blood).

Apart from Chisholm's considered reappraisal of the use of EDTA, a further concern is the discharging from hospital of Aboriginal patients on oral D-Penacillamine. Dr E Robertson (personal communication) suggests that if an Aboriginal patient were to continue to inhale leaded petrol while taking Penacillamine, then lead absorption would be increased. There is no sure way of guaranteeing that an individual discharged from hospital will not recommence sniffing once in his or her home community. In the case of pica or exposure to other sources of environmental lead, it is much more feasible for physicians to recommend a course of chelation therapy and to take action to prevent continued exposure to contamination. In the case of petrol sniffing, this is simply not possible.

Notwithstanding these research findings and the uncertainty surrounding the use of chelating agents in the treatment of organic lead intoxication, researchers and hospital physicians alike take the view that chelating agents may have possible beneficial actions. They are used also because no other antidote is known (Grandjean 1984, 236).

NOTES

1. The United Kingdom Department of Health and Social Security report 'Lead and Health' notes ingested lead absorption to be an average of 11 per cent with 'a very wide absorption rate among adults...the absorption factor is not constant, even for an individual, and depends upon such factors as amounts of fat, minerals (particularly calcium) and vitamins' (Department of Health and Social Security 1980, 44). One theoretical study showed that the increase in blood lead concentration per 100 micrograms per day of lead in the diet would be 3.6 micrograms per decilitre of blood (1980, 45). See Moore (1980, 334) for figures on pulmonary absorption of lead.

2. The reference range for blood lead levels used by the Northern Territory Health Department is as follows: 2.05–2.35 micromols of lead per litre of blood = possible exposure; 2.4–3.8 micromols of lead per litre of blood = possible toxicity; 3.85 micromols of lead per litre of blood = lead poisoning.

3. I am grateful to Chris Burns, Armidale College of Advanced Education, New South Wales, for drawing my attention to Chisholm's article.

CHAPTER

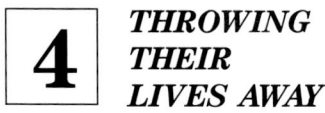

4 THROWING THEIR LIVES AWAY

In an extensive search of the medical literature, Grandjean found about 150 fatal cases of organo-lead poisoning in seven different regions of the world, most of which were industrial exposures. He notes only one fatality (in 1978 in the United States) from gasoline sniffing (Grandjean 1984, 229). In Australia, the official figure for deaths associated with the inhalation of petrol fumes is twenty in the nine years from 1980 to 1988 inclusive (National Drug Abuse Information Centre 1989). We can assume that the majority of these fatalities were Aboriginal. In New Zealand, the deaths of eight petrol sniffers have been officially reported between 1977 and 1986 (see Table 4).

DATA ON ABORIGINAL DEATHS

The question of Aboriginal petrol-related fatalities is an emotive one, exacerbated by the proliferation of media reports and anecdotal accounts in recent years. Several witnesses to the Australian Senate Select Committee on Volatile Substance Fumes in 1985 mentioned instances of fatalities (Senate Select Committee, 211, 1280, 1380, 1414) and other published accounts provide scattered data (Smith and McCulloch 1986; Freeman 1985; Kaelen et al 1986). Perhaps as a result of the limited accurate data available at the time, and the seemingly low incidence of deaths reported in the Northern Territory, the Senate Select Committee did not emphasise mortality

Table 4: Deaths caused by petrol sniffing in New Zealand, 1977–1986

Year	Age	Sex	Race
1977	4	M	Maori
1979	15	M	Polynesian
1984	17	M	not known
1985	13	M	not known
1985	15	M	not known
1985	11	F	Polynesian
1986	13	M	Non-Maori
1986	15	M	Non-Maori

Total reported deaths: 8
(Source: National Co-ordinator on Solvent Abuse for New Zealand)

in its report (1985, 189–191). The time has now come to take sniffing-related deaths more seriously, and to examine in more detail the regional distribution of these fatal cases.

Because many earlier fatalities are so hard to validate, I propose to rely on three sources of mortality data. These are:

1. The overall figures compiled by the National Drug Abuse Information Centre in the Commonwealth Department of Community Services and Health. These are collected with the cooperation of all state and territory drug and alcohol authorities, whose staff search coroners' records. This collection is part of a national register of deaths from volatile substance abuse and of national forensic and poisoning case reporting systems (which monitor drug-caused sudden deaths and emergency ward admissions throughout the country).

2. The original, more detailed accounts obtained from coroners' records from which the above are drawn. With the cooperation of the Northern Territory Drug and Alcohol Bureau, the Epidemiology Branch of the Health Department of Western Australia, the South Australian Drug and Alcohol Services Council, and the Queensland Alcohol and Drug Dependence Services, I had access to extracts from coronial files on petrol-related deaths.[1]

3. Other data that I know to be accurate, which were collected by me from community clinic records or police reports. These data do not appear in either of the sources above.

Using the above sources, I compiled Table 5, which shows the documented deaths associated with petrol sniffing among Aborigines throughout the country between 1981 and 1988. This table shows the official cause of death and the number of years the deceased was known to use petrol. Table 5 details thirty-five deaths and shows that the majority of these reported fatalities occurred among males, only one female having died as a result of petrol sniffing in the eight-year period. The deceased were aged between twelve and thirty, the mean age being 19.22 years (see Table 6). Figure 6 shows the number of deaths by year; Figure 7 the number of deaths by the month of death. Seasons do not appear to influence the number of deaths.

Although coroners are becoming more aware of the relationship between petrol sniffing and causes of death such as pneumonia, it must be stressed that the figures provided in Table 6 are likely to underestimate the reality. For example, despite there being only one 'official' death caused by petrol sniffing in the Top End of the Northern Territory, some unofficial and anecdotal reports exist to suggest that other deaths have occurred (Senate Select Committee 1985,

Table 5: Documented deaths caused by petrol sniffing among Aborigines, 1980–1988

Year of death	Residence, state/territory	Sex	Age at death	Cause of death	Years used petrol	Source of information
1981	Bathurst Is., NT	M	19	pulmonary oedema caused by petrol inhalation	not known	NT Coroner's files
1981	Warburton, WA	M	17	burns (car accident while sniffing)	not known	WA Coroner's files
1981	Warburton, WA	M	16	burns (car accident while sniffing)	not known	WA Coroner's files
1982	Warburton, WA	M	14	general organ failure (car accident)	not known	WA Coroner's files
1983	Fregon, SA	M	30	inhalation of petrol fumes	not known	SA Coroner's report
1984	Warakurna, WA	M	12	shot himself while under influence of petrol	not known	Laverton police
1984	Laverton, WA	M	23	natural causes (chronic sniffer)	not known	Laverton police
1984	Cosmo Newberry, WA	M	13	not known (chronic sniffer)	not known	Laverton police
1984	Kalgoorlie, WA	M	25	cardio-respiratory arrest	at least 5	Kaelen et al (1986)
1984	Boulder, WA	M	18	accidental poisoning by petrol fumes	not known	WA Coroner's files
1984	Wingellina, WA	M	16	septicaemia (lower lobe pneumonia), depressed immune status from chronic addiction to petrol	not known	NT Coroner's files
1984	Amata, SA	M	21	septicaemia resulting from lung infection associated with petrol sniffing	'many years'	NT Coroner's files
1984	Indulkana, SA	M	17	poisoning by petrol vapour	'habitual'	SA Coroner's report
1984	Indulkana, SA	M	23	inhalation of petrol fumes	'some years'	SA Coroner's report
1984	Yalata, SA	M	20	cardiac failure caused by inhalation of petrol fumes	6	SA Coroner's report
1985	Tjirrkali, WA	M	20	inhalation of volatile hydrocarbons	not known	WA Coroner's records
1985	Warburton, WA	M	24	aspiration pneumonia	not known	WA Coroner's records
1985	Jameson, WA	M	27	not known (chronic sniffer)	not known	Laverton police
1985	Pipalyatjara, SA	M	19	non-traumatic petrol sniffing	not known	NDADS (SA)

Year	Location	Sex	Age	Cause	Number	Source
1986	Carpentaria Shire, Qld	M	18	toxic hepatic injury, probable petrol inhalation	at least 1	Qld Coroner's records
1986	Kalgoorlie, WA	M	17	pulmonary oedema resulting from petrol sniffing	not known	NT Coroner's records
1986	Mimili, SA	M	17	pneumonia, chronic lead poisoning and clinical lead encephalopathy	at least 4	NT Coroner's records
1986	Warburton, WA	M	20	chronic lead poisoning and broncho-pneumonia	not known	WA Coroner's records
1986	Warburton, WA	M	20	asphyxia caused by inhalation of petrol fumes and chronic lead poisoning	not known	WA Coroner's records
1986	Yalata, SA	M	19	respiratory arrest caused by petrol sniffing	8	Yalata clinic notes, via SA Coroner
1987	Warburton, WA	M	27	natural causes from self-neglect (demented state and numerous convulsions)	about 15	WA Coroner's records
1987	Wingellina, WA	M	22	asphyxia (food in larynx) brought on by petrol intoxication	at least 5	WA Coroner's records
1987	Coonana, WA	M	15	chronic lead poisoning and acute hydrocarbon toxicity leading to bronchial pneumonia	at least 4	WA Coroner's records
1987	Pt Augusta, SA	M	17	petrol sniffing	not known	NDADS (SA)
1988	Northam, WA	F	11	volatile hydrocarbon inhalation (lead in blood)	not known	WA Coroner's records
1988	Blackstone, WA	M	15	pneumonia and lead poisoning	10	WA Coroner's records
1988	Jameson, WA	M	19	pulmonary congestion pneumonia caused by petrol sniffing	'chronic'	WA Coroner's records
1988	Yalata, SA	M	16	cardiac dysrhythmia as a result of petrol inhalation	not known	NDADS (SA)
1988	Ernabella, SA	M	25	cardiac arrhythmia, myocarditis and chronic petrol inhalation	not known	NDADS (SA)
1988	Fregon, SA	M	21	cerebral effects of chronic petrol sniffing	not known	NDADS (SA)

Total deaths: 35

Notes on sources

NDADS (SA): National Drug Abuse Data System collection undertaken in South Australia by the Drug and Alcohol Services Council

Laverton police: Constable K Galton-Fenzi of Laverton police compiled notes on deaths associated with petrol not officially so attributed by the coroner, being privy to additional relevant details concerning the deaths.

Other known deaths associated with petrol sniffing (not noted above)
1979 Gerard, SA, 18-year-old male Aborigine (*Advertiser* April 1979, from coroner)
1983 Minto, NSW, 17-year-old male, race unknown (NSW Directorate of the Drug Offensive)
1989 Jameson, WA, 17-year-old female Aborigine (WA Working Party on Petrol Sniffing)
1989 Jameson, WA, 21-year-old male Aborigine (WA Working Party on Petrol Sniffing)
1989 Davenport, SA, 6 Aborigines in house fire started by petrol sniffers (*Sydney Morning Herald* 22 June 1989)
1989 Wagga Wagga, NSW, 3 non-Aborigines drowned after sniffing petrol (*Sydney Morning Herald* 30 August 1989)

Table 6: Deaths caused by petrol sniffing, by age groups, 1980–1988

Age group	Number of deaths
10–14	4
15–19	16
20–24	10
25–29	4
30–34	1
TOTAL	35

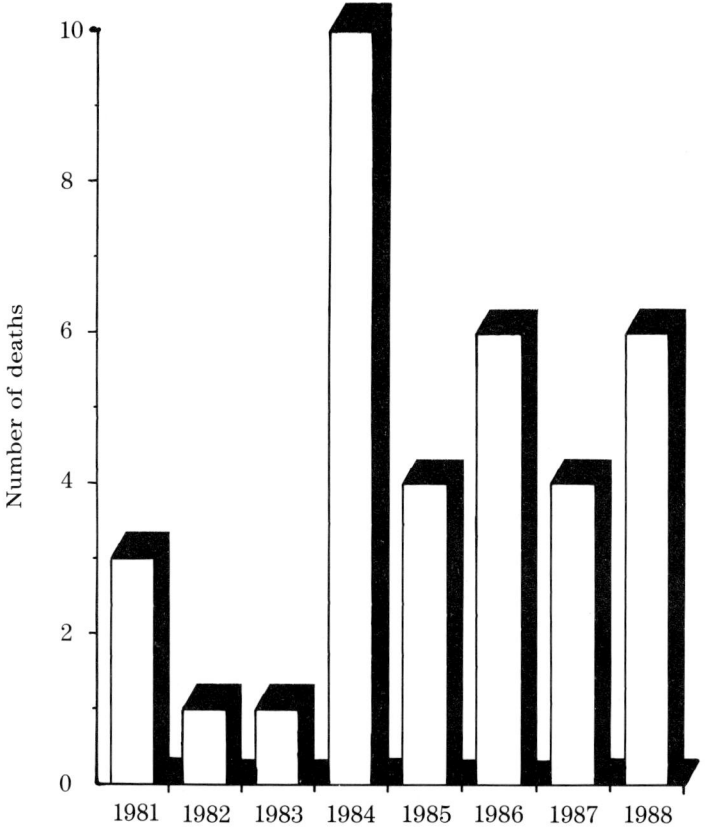

Figure 6: Aboriginal petrol-sniffing mortality by year, 1980–1988

1495, 1064).[2] Deaths of young Aboriginal men have been officially attributed to 'lobar pneumonia', for example, with no mention of petrol sniffing, even when the police have noted a container of petrol near the body (Dr A Smith, personal communication). I have included several deaths noted by Laverton (Western Australia) police to be strongly associated with petrol, but which do not appear in coroners' records as such. It is important that all facts surrounding a death are provided to pathologists conducting forensic examinations, and that copies of coroners' reports be forwarded to the home community clinic of the deceased, so that records can be accurately maintained, and the community members and relatives informed that a death was unequivocally caused by petrol.

THE DISTRIBUTION OF DEATHS IN AUSTRALIA

There appears to be a distinctive geographical distribution of the reported fatalities associated with petrol sniffing. It may be that the lack of uniformity in reporting procedures has produced this apparent geographical pattern, which therefore may not represent the real pattern of mortality. If we set aside the isolated instances

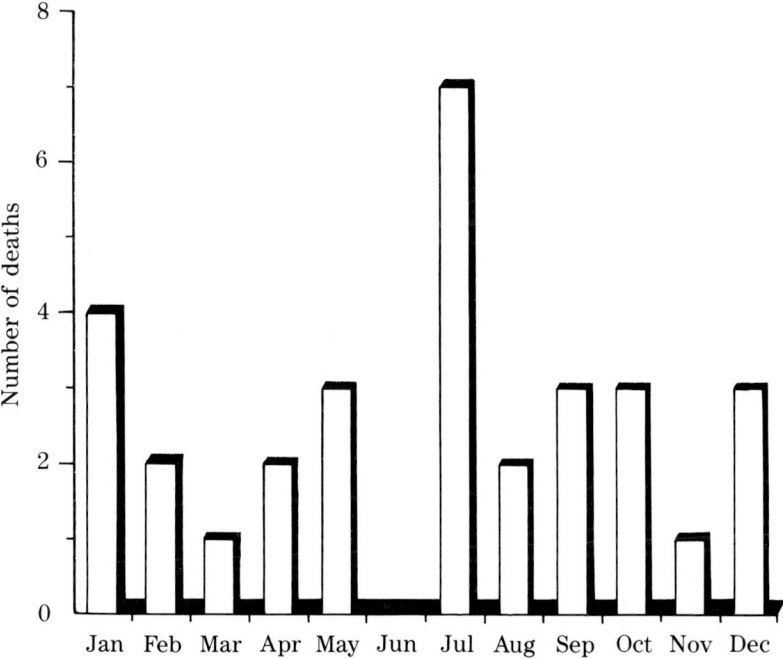

Figure 7: Aboriginal petrol-sniffing mortality by month of death, 1980–1988

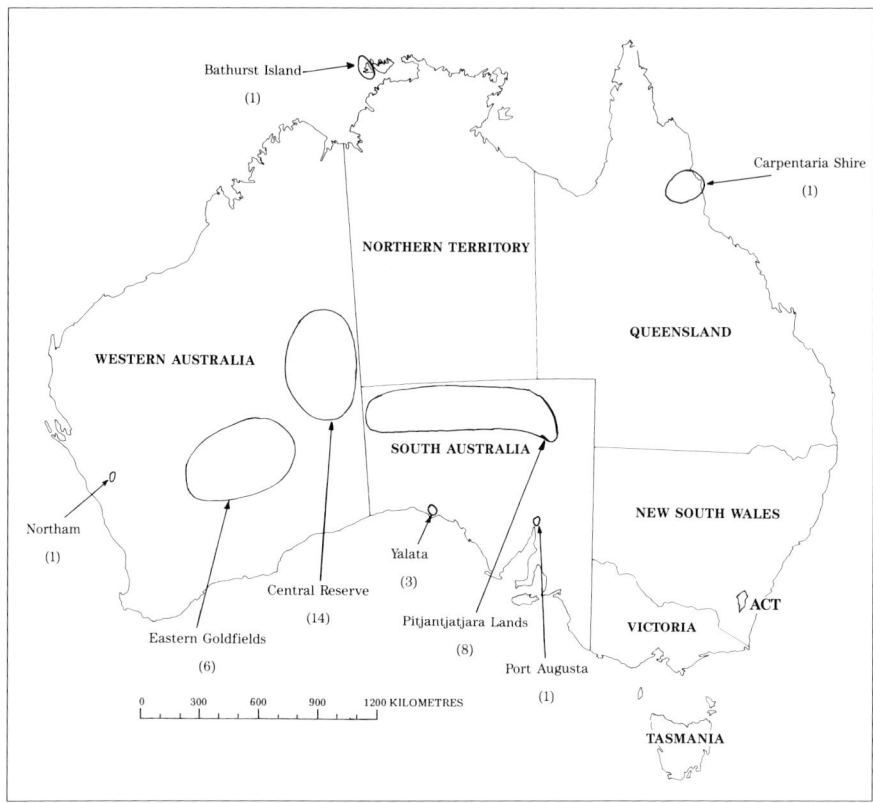

Figure 8: Distribution of deaths associated with petrol sniffing, 1980–1988

of single deaths in Queensland, in Western Australia (Northam) and in the Northern Territory (Bathurst Island),[3] we are left with a high number of deaths in what could loosely be termed the 'desert' regions of the country, from the north and far west regions of South Australia, across to the Central Reserves of Western Australia and southwest towards Kalgoorlie in the Eastern Goldfields region (Figure 8). In the other region of the country where petrol sniffing is common, parts of Arnhem Land and northern areas of the Northern Territory, only one death has been officially reported (on Bathurst Island) and that appears to have been an isolated incident, as petrol sniffing is not common on either Bathurst or Melville Islands. This anomaly deepens with the knowledge that petrol sniffing has been known to occur in Arnhem Land, and in the desert regions, for a similar length of time — approximately twenty years. Although there are fluctuations in use within communities — fluctuations that have been occurring over the last twenty years — there is no evidence to suggest that the overall prevalence of sniffing is necessarily diminishing in Arnhem Land as opposed to the Centre. Both regions have a similar age range of sniffers — from early teenaged adolescents to young adults in their twenties — and both regions regularly treat, evacuate and hospitalise sniffers who show symptoms of encephalopathy. What other reasons could there be for this regional difference, assuming that it is not merely reflecting differences in reporting?

We know from the published research that there are marked individual differences in the absorption of organo-lead compounds. Mahaffey (1985, 407) discusses the relationship between nutrition and lead toxicity (which I pursue shortly) and states:

> Humans have a physiological range in which adaptation to different external doses of a chemical is possible. When the combination of altered nutritional status and lead exposure occur together, the limits of adaptation are usually reduced. In clearly symptomatic disease a complex web of causation is typically present, but the most severe deficiency or toxicity tends to predominate.

Similarly, Grandjean (1984, 233) observes that several variables will affect the prognosis of someone with chronic lead intoxication:

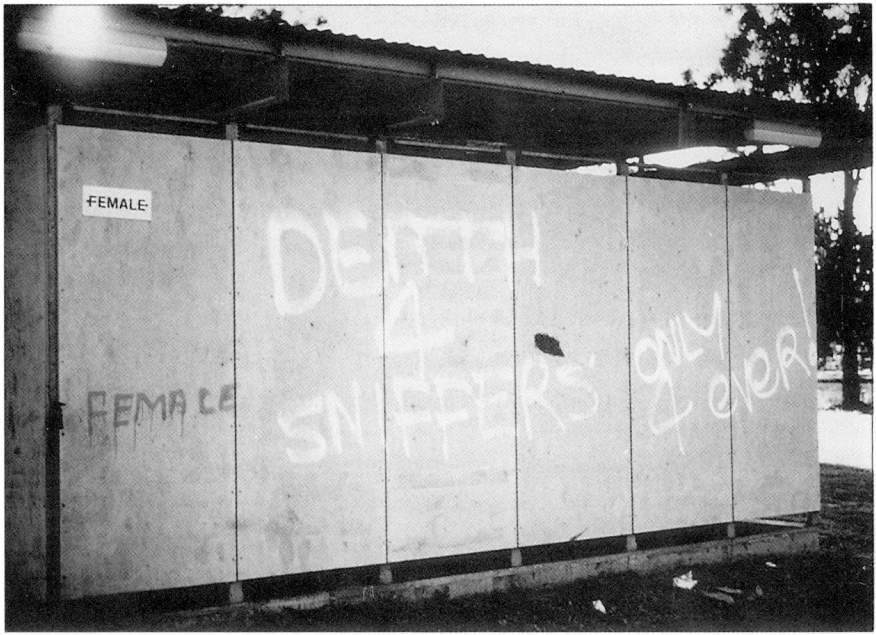

Plate 3: 'Death 4 sniffers' graffiti in east Arnhem Land

Aggravation may be related to increased exposure or to intercurrent disease, stresses, or non-specific factors. In some cases, a chronic intoxication may appear in a latent stage, subjective complaints being brought out only by special stresses, and the patient 'over-reacts' to other diseases.

If indeed there is regional 'vulnerability' to the toxicity of petrol among petrol sniffers, a variety of factors could be influencing their prognosis. One of these is individual susceptibility (as a result of general health status and nutrition); the other is the provision of health servicing and emergency care.

SUSCEPTIBILITY: THE ROLE OF NUTRITION AND HEALTH STATUS

There is evidence that nutritional status can influence an individual's susceptibility to the effects of inorganic lead, and that diet can influence his or her response to ingested lead.[4] It is unclear whether nutritional status is as important in the case of inhaled organic lead. It is perhaps useful to review some sources on the topic. The association between lead toxicity and nutrition was realised over a century ago when milk was used as a dietary supplement for lead industry workers to 'protect' them from lead poisoning. An individual's diet and nutritional status influence not only his or her absorption of lead, but also modify the toxicity of any external exposure to lead. Additionally, lead exposure can affect the utilisation of nutrients in the body (Mahaffey 1985, 390). Research on these factors has produced findings from both animal and human subjects, and is reviewed by Mahaffey (1982, 1985). I have drawn from her overview in the following discussion.

Researchers have found that the overall patterns of food intake can influence the absorption of lead. In other words, fasting or an erratic food intake serve to increase the absorption of ingested lead. This emerged from a Washington DC study of children of low-income groups whose food consumption fluctuated according to the arrival of social support payments.

Mahaffey mentions calcium, phosphorus, iron, zinc, vitamin E and dietary fat as being influential in the development of lead toxicity. She found that a low calcium diet increased susceptibility to lead toxicity approximately twenty-fold in animal experiments, and that low calcium diets also facilitated the accumulation of lead in the femur and the kidney. Studies of lead-burdened children have shown that children with elevated body stores of lead have a lower dietary calcium intake. Phosphorus deficiency will increase susceptibility to lead toxicity, as will iron deficiency, which is known to be far more common. If indeed these nutritional factors are important for those who inhale lead while sniffing petrol, then Aboriginal nutrition may be a cause for concern. The Nganampa Health

Council environmental and public health review of Anangu Pitjantjatjara Lands (1987, 64, 69) in northern South Australia notes:

> The diet is high in energy, very high in refined carbohydrate, high in fat and salt and very low in dietary fibre. This pattern of dietary intake is consistent with obesity and associated conditions... . Intake of most vitamins and minerals is inadequate. Diets are commonly low in A and B vitamins, especially folic acid and B6 and frequently zinc and magnesium.

There are variations in dietary intake and nutritional status both within and between Aboriginal communities, as pointed out by Cowlishaw (1982a), Harrison (1986) and Lee (1988). These variations are caused by a number of factors, including the ecology of the region, seasonal changes, the remoteness of the community and the accessibility of facilities, store contents and turnover, mobility of residents and their access to bush foods, and gender differences.

The availability and variety of bush foods vary considerably between northern communities, where fresh and salt-water fish are plentiful, and desert communities, where animal flesh is the primary source of meat. People in both regions who engage in hunting for bush foods may consume huge quantities of protein from meat (O'Dea et al 1988; Palmer and Brady 1991). However, there are so many individual and community variables that affect the quantity and range of bush foods sought and consumed that it is virtually impossible to make generalisations. As a hypothesis, though, it can be suggested that for coastal or riverine Top End people, the availability and diversity of seafood, animal food and vegetable food are greater than the availability and diversity of bush foods hunted in desert regions. Whereas coastal and riverine people always have such foods available to them if they want to seek them out, in several desert areas kangaroo and turkey may be seen rarely, or may require many hours of labour to obtain. Observation suggests that, whereas northern groups still consume a wide variety of vegetable foods (yams, roots and fruits), the range of vegetable foods still consumed in the desert may be diminished. It is difficult to say whether there are marked differences in the nutritional status of northern and central Australian Aborigines. The potential impact of such status on the susceptibility of individuals in each area to the toxic effects of petrol is also pure speculation.

In conclusion, it can be stated that there is a demonstrated association between dietary and nutritional factors and susceptibility to the toxic effects of inorganic and ingested lead. It is possible that erratic diet and, in some cases, poor diet among Aborigines may influence the vulnerability of individuals to the toxic effects of organic and inhaled lead. In addition, we know that the respiratory system is vulnerable to the effects of volatile solvents. Repetitive inhalation of highly concentrated solvent mixtures may predispose individuals to bacterial and viral infections. Pneumonia and other lung infections are frequently observed in solvent abusers (Fornazzari 1988, 101). The abuse of petrol, which contains a variety of hydrocarbons, would be expected to exacerbate any pre-existing lung infection. Symptoms associated with lead or hydrocarbon toxicity can be aggravated by the presence of 'intercurrent disease, stresses or non-specific factors' according to Grandjean (1984, 233). Any or all of these factors may be influencing the mortality data for different regions in Australia.

EVACUATION AND TREATMENT OF SNIFFERS

Intoxicated petrol sniffers are difficult to manage in community clinics, and most community health staff seek to evacuate grossly disturbed patients to hospital. It is possible that a number of variables associated with evacuation and hospitalisation might be influential in the patients' prognoses, for example, some regions may be evacuating sniffers more readily and more frequently than others.

By analysing the log book of the clinic in one Arnhem Land community, Maningrida, it was possible to enumerate petrol-sniffing related evacuations from the community. Maningrida has an Aboriginal population which varies between 600 (in the dry season) and over 1,000 (in the wet season), a well-staffed clinic and a district medical officer who visits regularly. The number of people using petrol as an inhalant varies greatly and sniffing disappeared entirely for several months in 1988. From the reliable sources available, it is estimated that there are approximately sixty users of petrol at Maningrida. Of this number, twenty-five individuals have been evacuated to Royal Darwin Hospital over the five years from

Table 7: Hospital evacuations by individual and sex, Maningrida, 1984–1988

Sex					Total
Number of evacuations	1	2	3	4	
M	12	5	2	-	19
F	3	1	1	1	6
Total	15	6	3	1	25

1984 to 1988 inclusive (see Table 7). This means that approximately 41 per cent of petrol users had been evacuated over this period.

Most individuals were evacuated (and thus hospitalised) on one occasion; however, one individual was evacuated and hospitalised on four occasions. Fluctuations in the intensity of the practice over several years can be gauged to some extent by the number of evacuations (see Figure 9). In 1987, for example, the total number of evacuations for all reasons was 398, of which fifteen (3.8 per cent) were related to petrol sniffing. All evacuations from Maningrida are by air and are executed promptly (one and a half hours flying time from Darwin) by the Northern Territory aerial medical service.

Some evacuation data are available for people living in more central regions of the country from the Nganampa Health Council, which provides health services to the Pitjantjatjara Lands. The Aboriginal-controlled health council employs both medical and nursing staff who reside in major settlements on the lands. Most evacuations are by air although there is also road access. Over a period of eighteen months (1 January 1986 – 30 June 1987), forty-two individuals were evacuated for illnesses related to petrol sniffing. The estimated number of petrol users in the area serviced by Nganampa Health was at least 118 (Nganampa Health Council 1989, 46). This means that approximately 35 per cent of petrol users were evacuated as a result of their sniffing over this period. However, this estimation is complicated because it includes an atypical mass hospitalisation of petrol sniffers that occurred in the last quarter of 1986. Between 1980 and August 1985 there were sixty-five admissions to Alice Springs Hospital related to petrol sniffing, involving twenty-five individuals (Commonwealth of Australia 1985, 190).

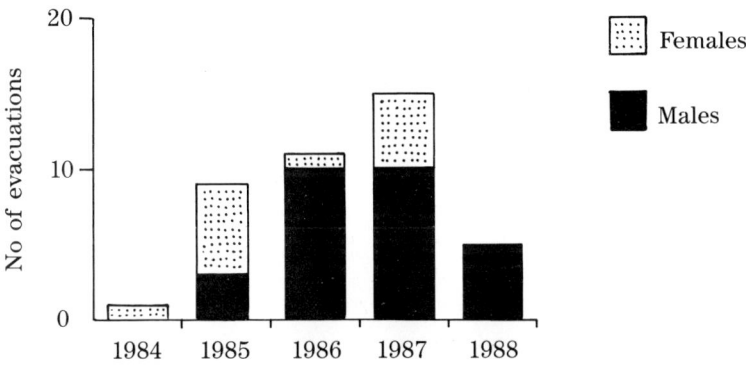

Figure 9: Evacuations to hospital from Maningrida for petrol-sniffing symptoms, 1984–1988 (figures from Maningrida community health centre)

Evacuation data were not available from Western Australia as the RFDS (Kalgoorlie) has not yet fully computerised its records. The policy of the RFDS at Kalgoorlie base has been changed recently so that aerial evacuation for petrol sniffers is now conducted only in situations designated as 'emergencies'. According to RFDS staff at Kalgoorlie (personal communication), this change in policy was said to have come about as a result of the number of hospitalised sniffers who absconded after a short period. Kalgoorlie base runs four aircraft, covering an area of 640,000 square kilometres, which extends from south of Kalgoorlie and northeast to the Central Reserves as far as Kiwirrkura (near the Northern Territory border). Transfers to Perth hospitals are also undertaken by RFDS. This reluctance to accept patients suffering from the symptoms of petrol inhalation means that the burden of their care rests with community-based health staff, often solitary nursing sisters in busy clinics. There are no medical staff resident in the settlements.

Bearing in mind the logistical differences (number of aircraft, distance, road access) between the servicing of the Central Reserves in Western Australia (now Ngaanyatjarra leasehold land) and that available to the Pitjantjatjara Lands and locations such as Maningrida in Arnhem Land, it would appear that evacuations, and thus hospitalisations, occur less frequently in Western Australia.

Apart from possible regional differences in susceptibility (as a result of health and nutritional status) and differences in the management and treatment of symptomatic sniffers, there are several other variables which should be mentioned. There are, for example, differences in the tetraethyl lead content of petrol between Australian states and territories. The Australian Institute of Petroleum provided the following current maximum permissible levels of lead in leaded petrol for each state:

Queensland	.84 grams per litre
Western Australia	.84 grams per litre
New South Wales (rural)	.84 grams per litre
South Australia	.65 grams per litre
Northern Territory	.65 grams per litre
Tasmania	.45 grams per litre
New South Wales (urban)	.40 grams per litre
Victoria	.30 grams per litre

According to these figures Western Australia has one of the highest maximum permissible levels of lead in Australia — up to .84 grams per litre, which is also the international permissible maximum. This does not mean that all petrol in the state contains this amount of lead, but such levels are permissible (R Corinaldi, Australian Institute of Petroleum, personal communication). Other variables that could potentially influence the extent and seriousness of petrol-related morbidity (and perhaps mortality as well) include such imponderables as the size of containers used by sniffers, the length and intensity of bouts of sniffing activity and the age at commencement of the practice.

In conclusion it is clear that the situation with regard to fatalities associated with sniffing is substantially different from what it was ten years ago. Perhaps as a result of better collections of drug-related mortality figures, and perhaps as a result of an increase in the habitual (rather than occasional) use of petrol as an inhalant over the last ten years, there are now a number of deaths occurring: my estimation is a minimum of thiry-five Aboriginal deaths between

Table 8: Deaths caused by volatile substances Australia-wide, by age, 1980-1988

Substance	Age (Years)					
	0-9	10-14	15-19	20-29	30+	Total
Aerosol sprays						
Hydrocarbon	—	2	—	1	1	4
Fluorocarbon	—	1	10	—	—	11
Other	—	1	6	4	4	15
Liquid petroleum gas	—	—	2	5	13	20
Petrol	—	—	11	7	2	20
Typing correction fluid	—	2	6	—	1	9
Natural gas	—	1	—	2	7	10
Lighter fluid or gas	—	2	5	1	—	8
Anaesthetics	—	—	3	6	4	13
Glues, etc	—	—	2	—	1	3
Thinners, cleaning fluids	—	3	2	—	5	10
Others	—	—	3	3	4	10
Total	—	12	50(a)	29	42(b)	133(c)

(Source: National Drug Abuse Information Centre)
(a) includes one death which involved both a fluorocarbon spray and a lighter fluid
(b) includes one death which involved both correction fluid and natural gas
(c) the actual number of deaths recorded was 131, see footnotes (a) and (b)
Aerosol sprays were the most abused substances and accounted for 24 % of all substances found; the 15-19-year age group alone accounted for 37% of all substances found; in the 30+ age group, liquid petroleum gas and natural gas accounted for 45% of all substances found.

1981 and 1988. The official Australia-wide statistics on volatile solvent deaths are provided in Table 8. The fact that many of these fatalities have taken place in particular regions, and are even clustered within particular groups of communities, concentrates the impact that these deaths have had on the small interrelated populations within which they occur.

NOTES

1. These data were collected with the assistance of Gloria Markey, Linda Hayward, Craig Faulkner and Grey Wrey in each state or territory.

2. These deaths were mentioned in a submission by Craighead, who notes (as a result of discussions with H Shepherdson, long-term resident of Elcho Island) 'several' deaths in the past. Dr HD Eastwell reports one 'well attested death' between 1978 and 1982 but provides no details.

3. Use of petrol was not common at Bathurst Island and petrol sniffing is not now practised there (J Devitt, personal communication).

4. Dr G Vimpani, Flinders Medical Centre, South Australia, drew my attention to the documentation on nutritional factors and lead toxicity.

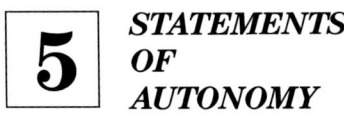
CHAPTER 5
STATEMENTS OF AUTONOMY

Well Friday and Saturday nights were just a, er, big...bore man, no scene, and all the other kids [at a Refuge] went out dancing, or out with Spunks [glue sniffers], and I was just crying all the time 'cos I was alone. Then Jacko, he's a real electric Abo Spunk said to me 'youze coming to Zoom?' I didn't know what it was all about y'know. But we all put in twenty-five cents and he came back with the Knocker from the Newsie and he put in a paper bag, y'know, ready to chuck, and y'know I still didn't get it, and well I didn't want to do it at first, but they were real Top Spunks, y'know, and when I started zooming, fuck....Wow! just spooked all my arms and legs, like unreal...man. ('Cheryl', sixteen years, in Mills 1986, 11)

In the typology proposed by Norman Zinberg (1984), there is a close interrelationship of set (personality/individual motivations) with the setting (social context) variables in any understanding of drug use. As a result of the emphasis given to external factors (poverty, discrimination and cultural oppression) in the study of the causes of drug and alcohol abuse among Aboriginal people, the individual's motivations and perceptions have been neglected, and an important perspective has, as a result, been lost. This chapter explores some reasons for petrol sniffing among the Aboriginal people I worked with in several regions. Leaving aside the question of whether young people who choose to sniff petrol are somehow differentiated (by deprivation or family dynamics) from other young people, I sought to gain an emic (an insiders') perspective on explanations for sniffing. In seeking such an understanding, I avoided focussing solely on users of petrol themselves, being mindful of the difficulties of being seen to take an inordinate interest in their actions. Although I spoke with sniffers, I also interviewed ex-sniffers, as well as close family members.

EXPLANATIONS AS STRATEGIES

In the course of my research many non-Aborigines offered me general explanations for the abuse of petrol. Franks and the petrol-sniffing prevention team with which she worked had the same experience (Franks 1989, 20):

> Some service staff could not let go of old ideas that were simple solutions that were service-oriented and managed. We encountered the 'nothing-but' syndrome: 'petrol sniffing is

nothing but boredom — search for excitement — culture shock — poor nutrition, etcetera'.

Another series of explanations was offered by Aboriginal people. It was suggested variously that sniffers' parents spent too much money on alcohol; that they did not know how to bring up their children properly; that a sniffer had been spoilt as a child and so on. On some occasions people frankly admitted that they did not know why children sniffed petrol. Aboriginal people exposed to some church-based intervention programs which subscribe to the disease model, express the view that children who sniff (like adults who drink to excess) are sick. Many of these suggested reasons reveal that, to some extent, Aboriginal people have begun to adopt non-Aboriginal perceptions of deviant behaviour, a phenomenon that social scientists have noted elsewhere. Kunitz and Levy (1974, 255) discuss the changing definitions of substance use among Navaho Indians, suggesting that a society in the process of redefining itself comes to consider certain groups as deviant.

> As the society changes, however, these behaviours increasingly come to be seen as maladaptive to the new world where people are expected to be at work on time...where all sorts of obligations to the dominant society must be fulfilled. Many of these behaviours which were not necessarily disruptive or maladaptive in the traditional society clearly are so now. In the new society...the drinker's behaviour comes to be defined as sick. He is no longer a man who drinks a lot; he is an alcoholic.

It is possible to interpret some emerging Aboriginal views about the use of petrol in a similar light. Whereas overt expressions of deranged behaviour were (and still are) often accommodated and tolerated, there is increasing pressure on Aboriginal community members to perceive drunken comportment and exuberant sniffing as deviant and unacceptable (men should be at work, not drinking; children are supposed to be at school, not sniffing petrol). This pressure to redefine certain behaviours as maladaptive often emanates from Aboriginal para-professionals employed by government and non-government agencies, as well as from non-Aborigines.

Explanations offered by Aboriginal people, such as those noted above, can be interpreted as strategies whereby these people are attempting to come to terms with behaviours increasingly defined as 'deviant'. In order to make sense of events or actions perceived to be incomprehensible or disordering, all human societies develop strategies for explaining and accommodating these events. Such explanatory models, which may be derived from 'folk' theories about health and illness, constitute conceptual resources employed by individuals and communities

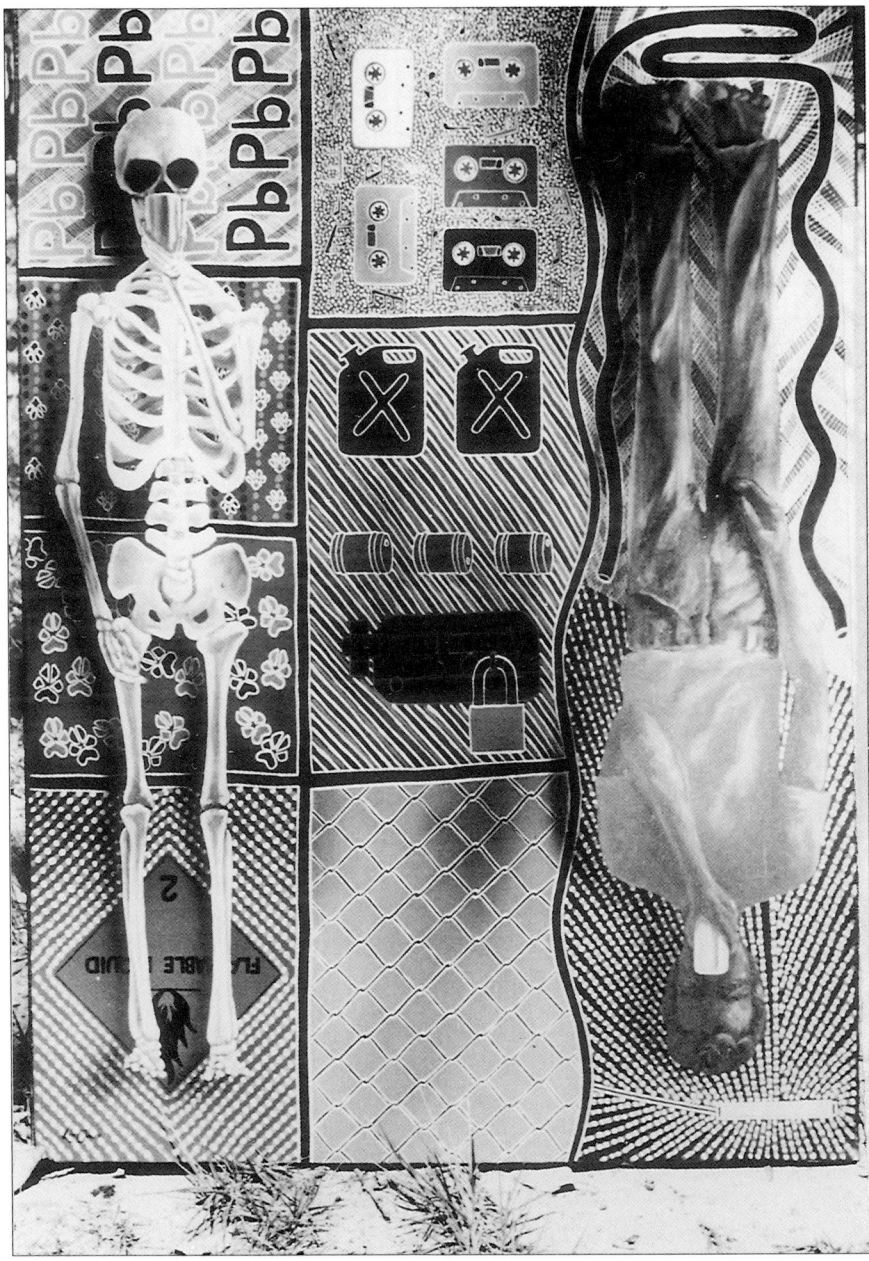

Plate 4: *Sniffer*, 1986, acrylic on canvas, 122 x 91 centimetres, painted by Victorian Aboriginal artist Lin Onus in an Arnhem Land settlement (reproduced with kind permission of the artist)

in order to cope with disruption effectively (Higginbotham 1984). The explanations for petrol sniffing offered by Aboriginal community members are, then, part of a repertoire of techniques for making sense of the situation. In addition, when these are offered to a questioner from outside the community, they become part of an 'official' or outward definition of social reality, supplied by informants who see themselves as spokespersons with a mandate from the group to present an account of itself.

AUTONOMY AND RELATEDNESS

Aboriginal social life, in the areas where I undertook my research, is marked by an emphasis on the autonomy of the individual, while at the same time it stresses notions of relatedness between people — connections that require constant outward expression through generosity, compassion and concern. Unrestrained generosity is understood by Western Desert and Arnhem Land people as an expression of love. The notion has been captured in the phrase 'caring and sharing' which is now featured in health education posters distributed to Aboriginal communities by the National Campaign Against Drug Abuse. Generosity is instilled into young children from a very early age, with older relatives urging toddlers to share highly valued commodities (usually chips and cool drinks) with others. Annette Hamilton's (1981, 151) work on child-rearing in Arnhem Land articulates most succinctly Aboriginal notions of indulgence and generosity:

> The reason for sharing...devolves around the notions of relationship and need, indicating that the one who has is obliged to give to the one who lacks as long as the latter indicates his desires... . By starting with the assumption that generosity is natural, it becomes so.

Fred Myers (1986, 113), working with Pintupi people in Central Australia, notes that training children to be generous is closely associated with the concept of compassion, of feeling sympathy. A child in possession of something desired by another is told to 'be compassionate and give it to him'. Indulgence is obligatory, as Hamilton (1981, 161) explains:

> The child is born with a set of needs, indicates these needs to others, and the duty of others is to respond; there is no difference for a small child between want and need, and...these things remain hard to differentiate throughout life... . [This model] denies that indulgence will produce selfishness and lack of sociability and asserts instead that indulgence is the right of everyone when a child, and indulgence is the duty of everyone when adult.

The extent to which people share is also an indication of the value people place on their relationships; it shows whether the individual considers a relationship to be important (Myers 1986, 115). Someone who is not generous is called 'hard' by Western Desert people; among Pitjantjatjara speakers at Yalata, South Australia, European staff who overtly refused Aboriginal requests or who berated people were said to be *witu-witu* (hard, unyielding). Giving freely, then, is synonymous with an expression of love, care, concern and compassion for another, and people must be subtle in their deflection of excessive demands or else face accusations that they do not 'like' the person refused or that they deny the relationship. A mother is required to accede to the demands of her children, to show generosity, and tries to avoid being seen to cross them. An early ethnographer (Warner 1969, 87) who worked in northeast Arnhem Land described this relationship:

> There is constant tribal pressure on a mother to be good to her children. No Murngin[1] mother would dare correct her children in the manner of a European woman, for she would be considered cruel and inhuman. Camp gossip and opinion would uniformly condemn her and liken her to an animal. On the other hand, there is less restraint on a son and daughter concerning their mother than in our own society. They frequently curse her.

Young people are treated as autonomous individuals, and learn from an early age that they have a wide range of freedoms — a much wider range than would be tolerated by most white Australians. Children learn the hard way, by experimentation and through freedom to explore. I have watched young children playing with fire in increasingly daring games, jumping on the fragile roofs of deep rainwater storage tanks, and sitting at the controls of moving vehicles, without intervention from adults. Risk-taking is an important feature of these exhibitions of exuberance and autonomy.

As with children everywhere, Aboriginal children need cajoling and persuasion to make them accede to the demands of adults. Many Aboriginal adults give up with a laugh and a shrug of the shoulders after trying to impose their will. Hamilton, among others, observed the tantrums and aggression directed towards mothers who did not give children what they wanted, or who tried to make them act against their wishes (Hamilton 1981; Myers 1986; Harris 1984). Reviewing the literature on socialisation and parenting, Cowlishaw notes several authors who comment that boys are even less subject to the mother's discipline than girls, and that their behaviour is uncooperative and often hostile towards her. If she castigates a boy, she will often incur her husband's anger. Citing Catherine Berndt, Cowlishaw notes that women lacked firmness towards children and showed indecisiveness even when it came to excluding them from a women's ceremony. Berndt also noted their submissiveness and lack of independence in their relationships with men (Cowlishaw 1982b, 498). Even after a boy becomes a 'man' at initiation, he could still make claims of food and demands for care from his mother.

The acceptance of personal autonomy and the unwillingness to impose one individual's will on another exists to such an extent in Aboriginal society that individuals are, at times, allowed to harm themselves, and to disrupt the flow of daily life for others. The toleration of potentially harmful activities and the requirements of generosity as an expression of caring extend beyond childhood socialisation into adult life. This means that the indulgence of children's wishes is another aspect of the indulgent attitudes to requests from all others (Cowlishaw 1982b).

Put simply, drugs enable individuals to exploit this finely balanced system. Drinkers of alcohol and sniffers of petrol (both groups predominantly male) are able to transform the notion of personal autonomy, and the emphasis on generosity and indulgence, to their own ends. At their disposal are communities of people who have been socialised into the belief that to refuse the direct request of a relative is tantamount to admitting that they do not care for them, and that to remonstrate or dissuade them from their drug use is to interfere with their right to do what they please with their own bodies.

Some examples from my research illustrate the ways in which young petrol sniffers exploit the 'loopholes' in what is, for the most part, a highly workable social system. Groups of sniffers exert pressure on their social milieu because their behaviour is unpredictable and frightening; the most common expression used by Aboriginal people is to say that they are 'wild'. A Pitjantjatjara man in a South Australian community explained sniffing thus:

> They want to make parents remember[2] them. 'If you won't buy anything for me, I can do anything!' If parents won't buy them clothes or food, tucker, if no food after school, no biscuits or chips, cool drink, mother says wiya ['no'], 'my parents don't worry about me' [thinks the sniffer]. They can talk back then.[3]

This speaker notes that sniffing is used as a manipulative or blackmailing device. Similarly, an east Arnhem Land woman, describing a young male sniffer, said he was 'proper no good; he is boss over mother and father'.

In Western Desert communities adults reported that petrol-sniffing youngsters exploit the generosity of relatives by demanding money or goods together with the threat 'You don't love me! I'll go and sniff!' This is just one of the many reasons why the kin of sniffers find it difficult to deal with them. The suggestion that the child will go and sniff because the parents 'don't worry' is both guilt-provoking and shame-producing. As such, the accusation cuts into the very heart of Aboriginal understandings of relationships. A second example also illustrates this point. In a Western Desert community in Western Australia, a fifteen-year-old boy, while sniffing petrol, smashed a component on the community's television receptor dish in a fit of unrestrained anger. Several hours later his elderly grandparents, with whom he lived, purchased a new BMX bike for him out of their pension money. They said they 'felt sorry' for him. A combination of notions of compassion and generosity converge as an explanation of the actions of the elderly couple who placated the tantrum of their grandson with the purchase of an expensive and highly valued commodity. Petrol sniffers are frequently referred to in Pitjantjatjara as *ngaltutjara* (someone deserving of compassion, a poor fellow). Sniffers are often thought of sympathetically rather that critically; they are *ngaltutjara* because something must be causing them to behave in this way (Brady 1985a). Feeling compassion, then, has a range of emphases from the entreaty that a child give another his cool drink, to expressions of sorrow for someone's unaccountable behaviour.

MY BODY, MY BUSINESS

In some Aboriginal languages the term for 'body' is synonymous with 'person'. For example, the Pintupi/Luritja dictionary explains that *yanangu* refers to people, body, and to reality as opposed to unreality (Keeffe 1989). Autonomy of action and the belief in the right to control one's own body are inherent in Aboriginal social life. Those momentarily deranged by the ingestion of drugs will assert that they have the right to do as they please and that no-one can stop them. Drunkenness is the most common context in which such assertions are made, perhaps because inebriation usually provokes some intervention, even if only at the level of remonstration, which in turn provokes a response from the drinker. In a discussion of drinking and resistance among Wiluna (Western Australia) Aborigines, Sackett (1988, 71) suggests that drunken individuals react, often violently, to attempts by others to order or control them. He provides several ethnographic examples to reinforce his assertion, including an incident where an inebriated driver was berated for his reckless driving:

> Hearing this the driver dove back into the car, loudly started it and proceeded...to spin a series of circles in the road.[4] This was brought to a halt by his slamming into an embankment and stalling the engine.... . After berating one another for a time...the driver indicated he was his 'own boss' and could 'drive any way I feel'.

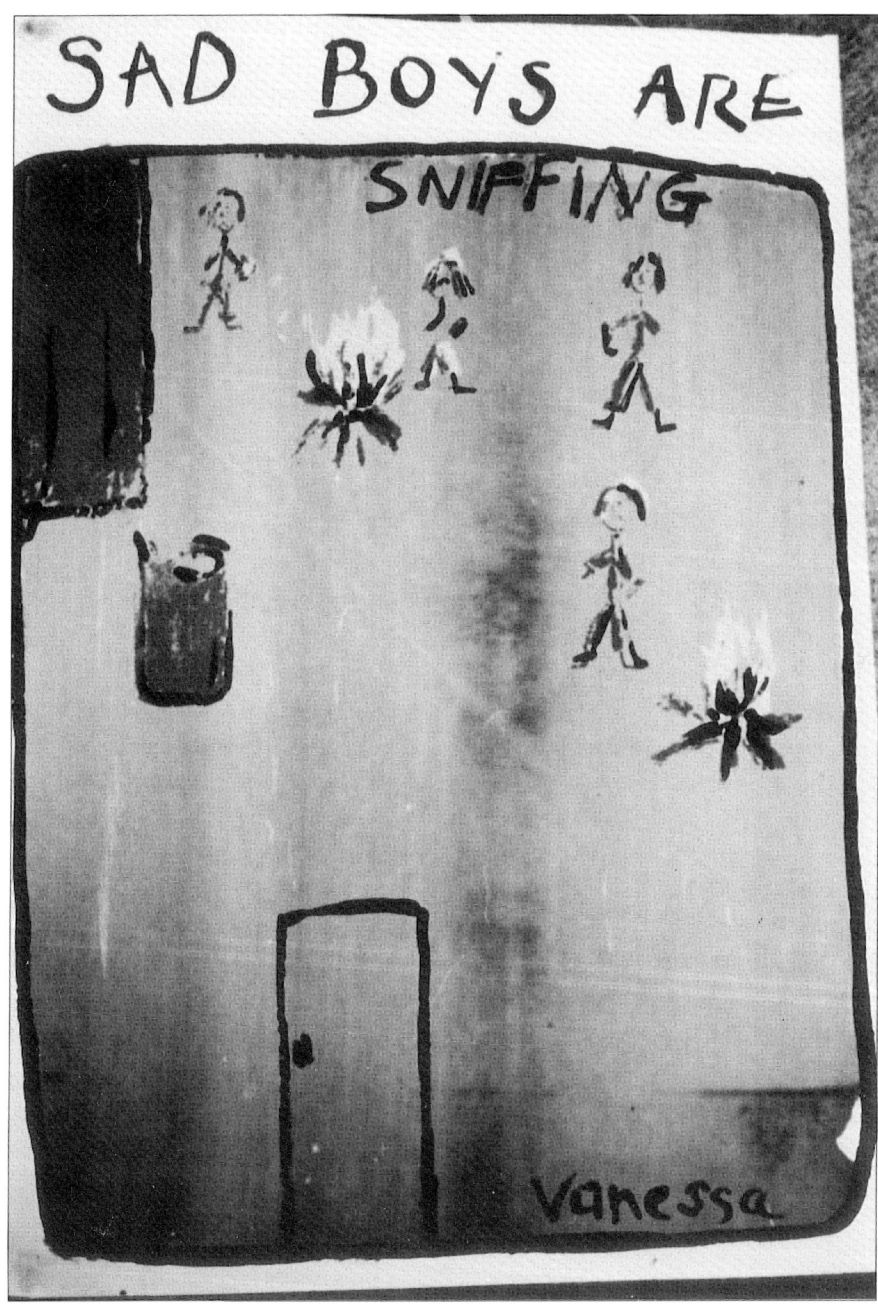

Plate 5: A poster by Vanessa Nampijinpa Brown from a competition at Yuendumu, 1984 (reproduced with the permission of the Aboriginal and Torres Strait Islander Commission and Hinton Lowe)

Drinkers resist the entreaties of wives and family members to desist, saying 'It's my own body, you can't stop me' (Brady and Palmer 1984, 42). Young people who sniff petrol show similar resistance to attempts to make them stop, and use identical arguments. Many family members have described how their interactions with sniffers met with a firm 'I'll do what I like! It's my body!' Grace Richards, a Warburton woman involved in a local petrol-sniffing working party, told me how she had asked her nephew why he sniffed. 'It's me', he replied, 'it's *me* sniffing'. Similarly, a young man in one community announced to some visiting whites that he 'sniffed juice'.[5] When one of the visitors began to indicate that this was not a very good idea, he quickly retorted that it was 'his business'.

In response to the exhortations of despairing family members, and of health education posters, that petrol sniffing can be fatal, some petrol sniffers retort that they want to die. Such statements raise the possibility that for some individuals chronic use of petrol is a form of suicidal behaviour, perhaps the ultimate expression of control over the body. In several instances where a death has occurred as a result of petrol sniffing, local residents have observed that the death had no apparent impact on the level of sniffing. This may be because of unwillingness to accept Western notions of the cause of death, but there is now a growing acceptance of the potentially fatal outcome of chronic sniffing, particularly in the desert regions where deaths have already occurred. We must assume that, among sniffers in communities where deaths of long-term users have occurred, there is some realisation of the role of petrol in the deaths. In an article on suicide and self-destructive behaviour among American Indian youth, Phillip May stresses that suicide rates vary tremendously from one location to the next, and over time. He also points out that suicide attempts were usually directed not at causing death, but at altering an important interpersonal relationship (May 1987, 62).

Whether or not it is valid to interpret long-term sniffing (with consequent severe symptoms, and repeated hospitalisations) as consciously self-destructive behaviour, it is undoubtedly the case that chronic sniffing has a number of impacts on close family members. They experience shame, guilt and embarrassment, anger and despair, and a sense of loss. Blame is levelled by some family groups against others whose children continue to sniff (Franks 1989, 16). In some cases, kin respond by withdrawal from the sniffer; in others, they respond by providing extra comfort and sustenance, taking the young person out bush on holidays, and to outstations in attempts to wean him or her off petrol. Either way, sniffing does provoke a response on the part of those close to the sniffer — an assertion that an individual 'wants to die' would be expected to provoke an increased level of response.

'GETTING SKINNY': ANOREXIA AND PETROL SNIFFERS

Anorexia, or loss of appetite, is frequently associated with petrol sniffing, both in medical research reports and in informal observations in the field. Aboriginal health workers, nursing staff in community clinics and the parents of sniffers all note that sniffers 'get skinny'. It has been assumed that sniffing itself is practised in order to numb hunger pangs (Ferguson 1978) and conversely that sniffing causes hunger (Morice, Swift and Brady 1981, 23). Eastwell suggests that 'hunger motivates the actions of sniffers when they become disinhibited, presumably because of increased activity without inflow of calories in the intoxicant' (1979, 222). Weight loss in association with petrol sniffing has also been documented in North America. A survey conducted in a Manitoba Indian reserve in 1987 found that 50 per cent of sniffers interviewed reported a significant loss of appetite and/or weight since they began sniffing regularly (Solvent Abuse Committee 1987, 12). It was, therefore, with some surprise that I learned that petrol sniffers in some Western Desert communities in Western Australia engaged in sniffing in order to lose weight. I quote below from three interviews which took place in three different communities in November and December 1988. The first person to alert me to this reason for sniffing was a young married man in his mid-twenties, an ex-sniffer.

> 1. [A friend] taught me how to sniff. I tried it and I liked it. It made me dizzy. I sniffed at Koonibba, at Port Augusta and Yalata. My uncle gave me a hiding and it blocked my nose. Then I got stuck into the grog. When you sit at home you eat all the time. When you sniff, you go for three or four days with no food, and then you 'see' food. It stops your appetite, eating. In Yalata, I never eat for a week — sniff and drink water. Got skinny. It shrink your brain and make your stomach skinny. Some like to sniff for the fun of it; some like to get skinny. I wanted to get skinny..... My sister-in-law comes in at midnight, steals my *mayi* [food] tin of meat. [She] sniffs on her own. She gutses herself and then sniffs more.

The second interview took place several days later and in another community in the vicinity of the first. Alerted to the suggestion that losing weight was a conscious aim, I asked about 'getting skinny' when I spoke with a mother of a petrol sniffer.

> 2. In the bush, they [sniffers] was good. After finish Law [ceremonial activity] they came home and sniffed. They tell lie, say they'll stop but don't. When everybody stops sniffing, they might stop. My daughter, she don't know sniffing, she only stop with mother right

through. W. [speaker's son] is *wati* [an initiated man] and he sniffs. He got healthy. He might think 'I don't want to be like my mother, big; I don't want to be woman'. So he sniff. They like to be skinny and bone. I've got a daughter short and fat, she don't sniff, she don't drink wine … . [My son] was watching pictures [hallucinating], getting frightened. I used to give him milk and raw egg and he got strong and he stop with me. Then he saw other lot they sniffing and he said 'that other lot, I might go'. Milk, because he was shaking. Every time I make tea with milk, get strong. Before when he was weak and shivering and frightened, I mix raw egg and milk. That petrol and milk was fighting and he used to run outside and I used to go and grab him and bring him back. Milk and eggs and he got better. He told me 'I wouldn't sniff' and he was a big healthy man, and then he said 'I don't want to be woman'.

The third interview took place in another community in the same region. This segment is extracted from a group discussion with four women who spoke about the sniffers in their region.

3. They like to get skinny. After all night sniffing, they sleep all day. Walk around all night. They skinny, they don't like to be fat. They shakes when someone hit them. They shakes a lot when they get hit from someone, nerves. So don't like to hit them because they'll die. When they sniff they go deeper and deeper, change face. Skin go in [the speaker pressed the skin on her cheeks in with her hands to demonstrate]. They don't go toilet, blocked. When they sniff juice, that tin get empty, like wine, go back, fill another one up. When not sniffing, they're dry. Sad face when not sniffing. White stuff come out from mouth — dry. They stay behind when families go hunting. They sit down and sniff behind.

As stated, these comments were elicited from people in communities of the Western Desert group in Western Australia close to the South Australian border. No similar comments were offered by Arnhem Land people in the Northern Territory to suggest that thinness was desired by sniffers, although Aboriginal health workers at Maningrida confirmed that weight loss occurs:

4. 'It's my body, you won't give me food so I'll sniff 'till I die' [the sniffers say]. Their brains get smaller, they don't think. Skinny, don't eat. It makes kids small, stay short.

Similarly, when a twenty-year-old woman who had given up petrol sniffing was interviewed, she spoke of food but not in the context of wanting to lose weight. The interview took place at a community in east Arnhem Land:

> 5. I make daylight, sniff 'till six o'clock in morning and went back home. Sometime it makes you hungry; my side [for me] it not. If I want to eat something else, fruit, if I was sniffing and I bin feel eating, dinner time I bin eat. Not much, I was really skinny. Twenty-four hours [I sniffed] I bin have maybe one bottle, two bottle petrol in my room and cordial bottle. Not this time, I bin Christian, I bin baptised and confirmed in river, I'm good life, health, getting strong and too much tucker.[6]

An account by an American native sniffer (Empowering Our People 1990, 1) reinforces the view that petrol sniffing is used deliberately by some to suppress appetite:

> I was always heavy set. I thought if I sniffed I would lose weight. I did. Also the music, there was always this music that I'd hear when I'd sniff. I wanted to keep hearing it.

How are we to interpret these statements? Anorexia nervosa is a syndrome treated by psychiatrists and behavioural psychologists in Western industrialised societies; it involves primarily highly motivated individuals, nearly all young women, who voluntarily and decisively starve themselves in order to achieve thinness. It is considered to be a disorder in which the patients' perceptions of their body images predominate — anorexics perceive themselves to be fat even when their bodies are excessively thin, even skeletal. It is also associated with the internal experience of lack of control, which in Western societies is felt more keenly by women than by men. Feminists interpret anorexia as a disorder brought about by the unhealthy conclusions some young women come to after seeing the slender female version of beauty portrayed in advertisements and fashion. Is it valid to interpret the desire for thinness among Aboriginal youth in conjunction with these views? Psychiatric analyses of anorexia nervosa often direct attention to the family of the sufferer, noting that the illness of the anorexic serves as a focus to bind together families on the verge of breakdown, and that the refusal of food and the deceptions associated with eating signify the assertion of control over the body, and over others. Finally, the medical literature tells us that the prognosis for anorexics can be extremely poor — once their weight is maintained at a consistently low level and the body begins to waste, death frequently occurs.

There have been few reported cases of clinically defined anorexia nervosa in the black populations of either Western or non-Western societies (Holden and Robinson 1988, 544). Anorexia nervosa is prevalent primarily among white teenagers in developed Western societies; there have been thirteen reported cases among American Blacks (Silber 1984; Pumariega et al 1984), and thirteen Black patients were seen at one London hospital between 1979 and 1985 (Holden and Robinson 1988).[7] There is only one reference to a case of anorexia in a developing country, Nigeria (Nwaefuna 1981) and there is certainly no reference to its presence among Aboriginal people in Australia. A compilation of four different studies of psychosomatic symptoms among Aboriginal communities by Eckerman et al (1984, 49) makes no mention of anorexia or eating disorders, despite covering categories such as somatic symptoms, anxiety, depression and insomnia. In a brief report of body-image among Arnhem Land Aborigines, Riley and colleagues reported that the majority of men and women were satisfied with their weight when asked whether they thought they were 'too skinny, too fat, or alright the way they were'. However, women were more aware than men of how their body weight compared to others in the community (Riley et al 1989, 88). Notwithstanding these findings, the statements I collected from Aboriginal people in both Arnhem Land and Central Australia made it clear that food has an important place in the discourse surrounding petrol sniffing (as indeed it does in discourses about other drug uses) (see Strathern 1987; Kohn 1987). It is sniffers' demands for food or the perceived withholding of food by family or friends that are said to be forms of emotional blackmail. It is through the provision of particular foods (milk, eggs) that women view themselves as helping their sniffing children become strong, and which serve to 'fight' the petrol. Women at Ngukurr (Roper River) in the Northern Territory also said that they had treated petrol sniffers by giving them milk. Explanations for the use of milk offered by these women were that it soaks up the petrol, it cleans out the insides, is good for digestion and promotes sleep, and that it helps sniffers to sober up.[8] One of the statements I collected indicates that a sniffer alternately gorges on food and then sniffs petrol. Each of the first three statements says unequivocally that sniffers do not like being fat, desire thinness, and achieve this through inhaling petrol.

Fatness and obesity are common among Aboriginal people in these desert regions and are associated by many researchers with dietary changes and a sedentary lifestyle — post-colonisation phenomena (Bastian 1979; Gracey 1977; Nganampa Health Council 1987). Surveys of sugar intake in Pitjantjatjara communities in northern South Australia found that people consumed up to the equivalent of sixty-six teaspoons of added sugar per person per day and three cans of soft drink per person per day (Nganampa Health Council 1989, 67). On the whole, leanness appears to be more common among Aboriginal people living in the tropics than among Central Australian Aborigines (O'Dea et al 1988; Riley et al 1989).

If sniffing to achieve thinness occurs as a response to the obesity of others in the community, then this explains why such motives were elicited from desert, rather than from Arnhem Land, people.

Among desert people, fatness is usually held to be synonymous with positive health and well-being, particularly in babies. Mothers in a Pitjantjatjara community where I worked smeared babies with echidna fat to make them strong and 'fat'. These people use the term *kanpi* (which means the fat of the emu and other birds) to refer to people and to signify well-being and happiness. 'Fatness' is desired of hunted animals. For Aboriginal teenagers using petrol it seems that fatness is associated by both boys and girls with femininity and being mothered, with sitting around at home and with eating. By getting thin through the practice of sniffing, Aboriginal adolescents are symbolically rejecting identification with family and with nurturing. They are taking control over their own bodies (by altering their body shape) but also exerting control over others (by deliberately counteracting the effects of nourishing food such as milk and eggs). By rejecting the sustenance offered by their parents and by becoming 'bosses' over their parents, they are, in effect, turning their culture on its head.

COMMENCING AND MAINTAINING USE

Several writers on drug use make the important distinction between antecedent factors that contribute to the commencement of use and those that contribute to the continuation of use. Miller and Ware (1989, 23–24) comment that:

> More recently, intrapersonal factors such as low self-esteem, anomie and locus of control have been posited as the most potent predictors of initiation. The available evidence, however, would suggest that a broad and complex range of personal and social conditions contribute to drug use and abuse.... . Additionally it appears that those factors that are related to the initiation of drug use may not be the same as those associated with continued use, problematic use, or abuse.

It is undoubtedly true that there is a 'broad and complex range of personal and social conditions' which serve to assist the drift into drug and alcohol use. The influential social conditions are, in the case of Aboriginal people, generally thought to be associated with social breakdown and dysfunction (Albrecht 1974; Kamien 1975). The personal elements have been interpreted as those in which drug use solves a problem, is a form of adolescent coping or provides users with the fulfilment of their desires, as well as achieving social or personal needs. In many cases, it is unlikely that the problems and needs of young adult and adolescent

Aborigines are very different from those of non-Aborigines of the same age. For example, United States researchers identified a set of social needs which, they argued, low-income black youth in Chicago shared with both their black and white counterparts in the middle classes. These are: positive self-image, personal dignity, ego enhancement and a sense of belonging and achievement. The black youths of whom they wrote met these needs through the elaboration of complex social roles involving gang-membership.[9] Perhaps there are fewer cultural differences between adolescents with different racial and social origins than is commonly thought. Women on Groote Eylandt, for example, said of their relationships with teenage sons:

> They sniff because their friends sniff. New generation, when they see friends sniff, they like to go and sniff. When they have problems at home, it makes them forget about problems. They think nobody cares, doesn't love them. I gave [son] belting and he said I hated him because of this...so I give him something to eat and not say anything when he come home. They say 'you don't stop people drinking or smoking', and 'it's our nature' .... [My son] used to sniff and he would say 'don't ask me, I'm tired'.... My little boy just ignored me, walk away. It makes us worry, nah.

The women who made these statements (which I have presented together) were frustrated and defeated by the behaviour of their children. One described how helpless she feels because her son is so miserable and unhappy. All are articulate, active women engaged in an adult education program in their community. They denied that children sniff because they are hungry or neglected, saying that the young people's groups share food and money among themselves, and that they (the adults) all tell their children they love them.

As with those starting to use many drug substances, petrol sniffers must be inducted into the mechanics and rituals of use. This is referred to universally by the Aboriginal people to whom I spoke as 'learning' to sniff — an expression bearing both a symbolic and a practical meaning. The passage from ignorance to knowledge of a substance is an important feature of Aboriginal social life, extending from the consumption of certain previously untasted foods to the ingestion of mood-altering drug substances. Some ethnographic data are required here by way of illustration.

Dealing with change and innovation has long been part of Aboriginal society, as people moved into new territory and received visits from outsiders. People learned of new foods available from the bush as they migrated, and incorporated new knowledge of the techniques of making such substances palatable. Naturally this process has gained momentum over the last three hundred years with the introduction of new substances from other regions — the Macassans brought rice, tobacco and alcohol to be shared with Aborigines across northern coastal regions. The Torres Strait Islanders, who drank kava in the early 1900s, had learned how to prepare the kava root by masticating and mixing it with saliva, and how to drink it out of half coconut shells (Chief Protector of Aborigines, 1911). The process of learning how to use a substance may require overcoming an initial distaste.[10] Women at Warakurna, Western Australia, told me that bush tobacco (*mingkulpa* in Ngaanyatjarra; *Nicotiana* sp.) was very strong: 'It used to make them sick when they first taste that wild tobacco. It make them sick up. Then lay down and next day…like that. Get used to it.' Even the consumption of bush foods is a learned affair, and it is said that children who have not tasted certain items have not yet 'learned' to eat them. In the Pitjantjatjara language, they are said to be *ngurpa* (unfamiliar) with these foods;[11] one who has tasted them is, on the other hand, *ninti* (knowledgeable). When people say that they are abstainers from alcohol or tobacco, they use the term *ngurpa*, saying that they have never learned how to drink alcohol or to smoke: 'I don't know drink'.

There is no difference between these conceptualisations and those associated with learning to use petrol. Sniffers learn how to sniff from their peers, from older users and from their siblings. Aboriginal people say that sniffing spreads from one community to the next because experienced sniffers 'show' or 'teach' the practice to others when they visit another place. 'Sniffing came from N', one person said, 'the boys from N came and showed them how to do it'. Aboriginal children are skilled at learning by observation and by imitation, since much of their socialisation is accomplished this way, rather than through receiving verbal instruction or explanation. Observing and witnessing are deemed to be synonymous with some transfer of knowledge or experience. Also significant in the context of petrol sniffing is the technique of learning by identification. Harris (1984, 78), writing of the 'crazes' for making shanghais or wheelies (tin trucks) among groups of boys in northeast Arnhem Land, says:

> There will be six or eight boys of ten or twelve years of age…often with an older brother of some of the boys leading the activity, but all busily watching each other work and then doing the same thing. Very similar mannerisms will be exhibited during the throwing of the spears to test them, or in the shooting of the shanghais, and these similarities come from the close imitation of elders or peers. It could be said here that learning is by identification, which is imitation of someone who is admired as a person. Learning by identification is very strong between sons and their fathers, or other older male relatives.

Certainly I noted that sniffers often had older brothers who were also users of petrol. In one family three brothers aged twenty-two, twenty and nineteen were regular sniffers and their younger twelve-year-old brother had begun to sniff. The prevalence of imitative behaviour has been noted among Aboriginal children in the form of 'crazes' or certain games and activities. Although many games, such as marbles and playing with toy trucks and shanghais, attract a constant level of attention from children, there are certainly high points in the popularity of some activities. 'Kung Fu' kicking games, home-made drum kits and breakdancing are examples. It is extraordinary that some observers should interpret this delight in doing what everyone else is doing as being pathological (see Cawte 1988); children and adolescents in the wider Australian society also become obsessed by passing crazes.

While induction into petrol sniffing is commonly referred to as 'learning' to sniff by Aboriginal people, abandoning the use of petrol is referred to as 'forgetting'. This expression does not literally mean they do not remember how to sniff, but suggests that an individual becomes unaccustomed, gets 'out of the way' of doing it. In Pitjantjatjara, people used the term *ngurparinganyi* (becoming unfamiliar). But the loss of familiarity with petrol sniffing can be tenuous, and sniffers may require only a trigger to 'start them all up again' as one person put it. This revival of an earlier familiarity is also referred to by Aboriginal people as 'learning'. The chairman of an east Arnhem Land community said:

> Before, boys and girls were not sniffing, they were playing volleyball and basketball. But now X came out of gaol and learned them how to sniff again. Boys and girls are sniffing.
>
> It was good here, our children weren't sniffing [as they had done in the past]. But then we went to G for thanksgiving and they saw them sniffing and [because they saw them] they came back here and did it. ...They were doing very well with the recreation but then some boys started acting silly and started them all up again.

From this discussion, we can surmise that there are two aspects to this concept of learning to sniff. The first is the initial exposure to a demonstration of the practice (and the actions that follow intoxication), but not everyone who observes sniffing acts upon that knowledge. This initial learning may be accompanied by induction into the paraphernalia and rituals of the substance use, discussed shortly. The second aspect of 'learning' to sniff follows a period of 'forgetting', when other activities overtake petrol use; it constitutes a refamiliarisation with the practice. Already previously inducted into the practicalities of use and having experienced the mood-altering effects, the user is reactivated (as it were) by identification with another (usually someone who re-enters the social arena of the community after a period of absence), and so takes up the practice once more. In these instances, interest in the substitution of other activities and pursuits is simply not felt keenly enough to maintain the period of abstinence.

When the initial learning takes place, new users learn what to expect when 'high', how to accentuate and enliven the experience, and they are introduced to the logistics and technicalities of administering the drug. A young woman from Groote Eylandt explained:

> My brothers were learning me how to sniff, [how to] get the tin, scrape the tin on cement to get top off. They taught me. It was killing my brain and the petrol bin go all over my body and I bin sick... . After that I was stealing too much, sniffing twenty-four hour... . Because I bin used to it, I make daylight, sniff till six o'clock in morning.

The speaker refers to a method of making a sniffing receptacle adopted over a wide area of Arnhem Land. By rubbing the end of an empty aluminium soft drink can on concrete, a user can shear the top off cleanly, so that the edges of the can can be squeezed and shaped to fit closely around the user's nose. The presence of piles of scattered can tops that have been removed in this manner signifies that petrol sniffers are active in the community — middens of can tops. Cans are sometimes elaborately worked and highly personal. Fanta cans are favoured in some communities, Coke cans predominate in others, and some are crimped with pliers down the length of the can to provide a convenient handle. In desert communities cardboard fruit drink containers are used as well as cans. The top-rubbing technique has not spread to these communities, so can tops are removed by using a knife or an axe. Supplies of fuel with which to top up the cans are often kept in two-litre plastic soft drink bottles. The more flamboyant sniffers tie these bottles to their belts so that they may replenish their cans and announce to all that they are determined sniffers of petrol.

Sniffers apparently enjoy the sensations achieved when high. These constitute part of the shared ritual of sniffing. It was thought enjoyable and fun to get 'the horrors', which is how hallucinations are described by sniffers in the Northern Territory. The following is typical of the attitude to the 'horrors', and was described to me by an ex-sniffer:

> When I was sniffing first, I had horrors...snake, ghost or devil, dog, animals, try to bite you, chase [you]. My favourite horror only snake. [Sniffers] do it to make feel strong. Start from

morning, maybe afternoon or night then you get a picture of a snake, animals. It make you feel funny way.

'Sniffers do it to make feel strong' — this statement was reinforced by a group of sniffers in east Arnhem Land who said that when they have sniffed petrol, they sometimes sit around a lighted candle, waiting for the Devil to appear. The Devil is expected to appear when the candle goes out. One boy admitted that he had stopped doing this because it was too frightening.

The mother of a sniffer described what happens to him when he sniffs, in an interview in a Western Desert community in Western Australia:

> They can see anything from that eye, [like] drive-in pictures. They close their eye and sniff and look at pictures. Cowboy, spider. Sometimes they chuck petrol and run when they see something — devils chasing them round — like [a] cat can be a big monster. They laugh at people. They see us different. They can see right through clothes, naked, when they look at people.

I quote these examples because they stress the actual experience of sniffing, and its appealing aspects — risk-taking, excitement, danger and access to a different world. These phenomenological aspects of sniffing are often neglected in the literature on aetiology, so that the reality of the act itself is lost. The individual experience of sniffing serves to perpetuate the drug use — the user wishes to re-contact the experience. Once inducted into the rituals of use and having experienced the 'horrors', the user becomes accustomed to these experiences. In Aboriginal English this is expressed as 'getting used' to a substance. This phrase occurred in a variety of contexts. The woman who spoke of initial reactions to bush tobacco said that those who chewed it 'got used' to it after they had been sick at first. Discussing the history of contact between Aborigines and missionaries at Warburton, Western Australia, an elderly man described the attractions of white people's food saying, 'We come around for lolly. We never knew bread or jams; we liked that bread and red one jams. We get used to it, get learn'. A final example of this process concerns an ex-petrol sniffer, who described how she came to sniff twenty-four hours a day 'Because I bin used to it, I make daylight, sniff 'till six o'clock in morning'. 'Getting used' to petrol, then, marks the transition from commencement of use to a habit of use.

GANGS AND HEAVY METAL

> Heavy metal music is basic music: loud, fast, dirty and arrogant. It's so dirty that if we moved next door, your lawn would die ('Hot Metal' in *Weekend Australian*, 19–20 August 1989).

In many communities, the groups of sniffers take on a decidedly 'oppositional' style, in which they cultivate the differences between themselves and mainstream Aboriginal society. This attitude, along with the ambience of danger and excitement associated with sniffing, helps to explain why new recruits are inducted into the practice. Sniffing offers an alternative to an unaided passage through the difficult years of adolescence and young adulthood and, as the women's comments presented earlier reveal, the sniffers shrug off their mothers' concerns. As one man said of the sniffers, 'I think they're just proud of themselves. "We don't listen to anybody", they say.'

If these are some of the reasons stated by Aboriginal people themselves for the commencement of sniffing, what are the reasons given by Aborigines for maintaining this drug use? The answer lies, at least in part, in the pleasures of the group. Over the last ten years, keen observers have commented on the rise of adolescent gangs notably in Arnhem Land (rather than in the Centre) (W Hastings, personal communication). These named gangs are still much in evidence in central and eastern Arnhem Land communities. 'We're the PS gang!'[12] three sniffers announced to me while we chatted. 'We like sniffing — it's fun, makes you mad, and you get horrors, like snakes chasing.' Other gangs were called

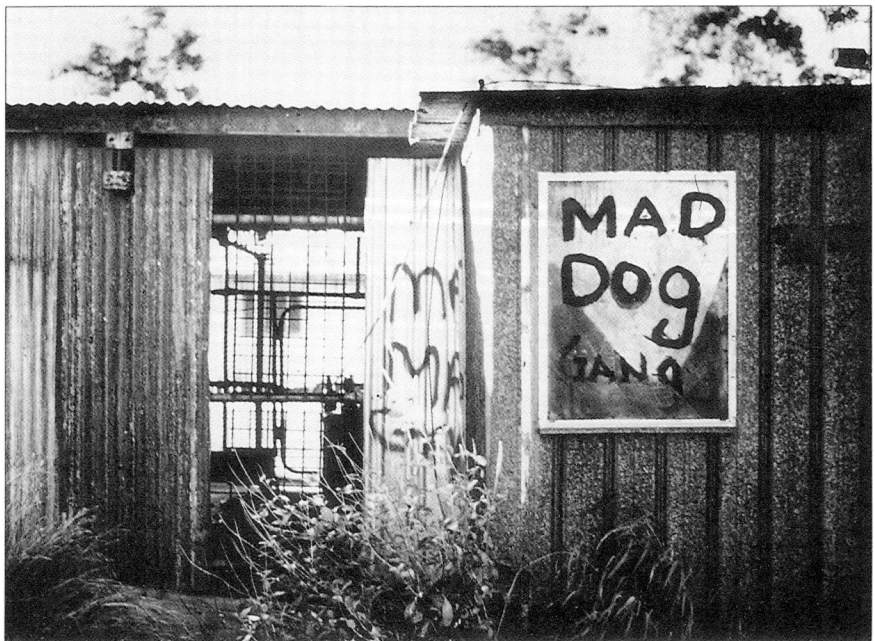

Plate 6: Mad Dog Gang graffiti in east Arnhem Land

the Skeletons, the Wongs and the Warriors, together with the German Rebels, Super Huns, Bad Brothers and Mad Dogs. Three girl gangs were said to be the Runaway Girls, Footloose and Lizhiz gangs. The Warriors and the Bad Brothers exist in other regions of the Northern Territory; in north-central Arnhem Land there was also the Spit Gang.

The gangs vary in their activities and reputations. A fifteen-year-old east Arnhem Land boy told me that the German Rebels (to which he belonged) did not get into trouble and had a territory of their own on the beach, where they had a shed for the older boys to stay in. Nevertheless, he said, they fight about 'anything'. 'We always get cheeky. We fight with arrows, we make arrows, spear. We fight in the long grass [between the houses and the beach] inside, where no-one can see.' The Wongs were thought to be the toughest gang and members carried knives and wore cordial bottles full of petrol around their necks. The supremely masculine ambience of the gangs has been partly inspired by the burgeoning popularity of videos, which is particularly prevalent in Arnhem Land. Virtually every house has a video machine; one I visited had three television sets. Kung Fu movies continue to fascinate these boys, although the Rambo films have now superseded them. A central Arnhem Land man told me that

> Sniffers have 'armies' in their fantasy, always have that armies in his or her mind and when they start sniffing, the other armies come and visit them and their own army does battle for them. Some kind of spirit controls them. Sometimes they lose and sometimes they win. They fantasise what they want to be in their own mind — just normal when not sniffing, no fantasies. Fantasies about being a War Lord, like in China, for their own group.

Gang membership is displayed by boys wearing T-shirts emblazoned with their gang name on the back (written on with felt-tip pens) and by graffiti which announce gang names and denounce other gangs. The Wongs had spray-painted their name on the reverse of a school sign. The Spit Gang had contributed their name to a more professionally drawn mural of a clown on the school walls. The gangs rise to, and fall from, prominence over time, and not all involve petrol sniffers. Their bow and arrow activities appear to be low-key by comparison with the Rascal gangs of Port Moresby, but their choice of gang names is remarkably similar in flavour to their Papua New Guinea counterparts.[13]

Another notable feature of this oppositional culture is its differentiation from the mainstream by way of attire. The youth of these Arnhem Land settlements, who have identified themselves with the separatist mores of the gangs and the petrol sniffers, wear decidedly different clothing and adorn their bodies in distinctive ways. Young men in these circles wear bandaids[14] on their faces and

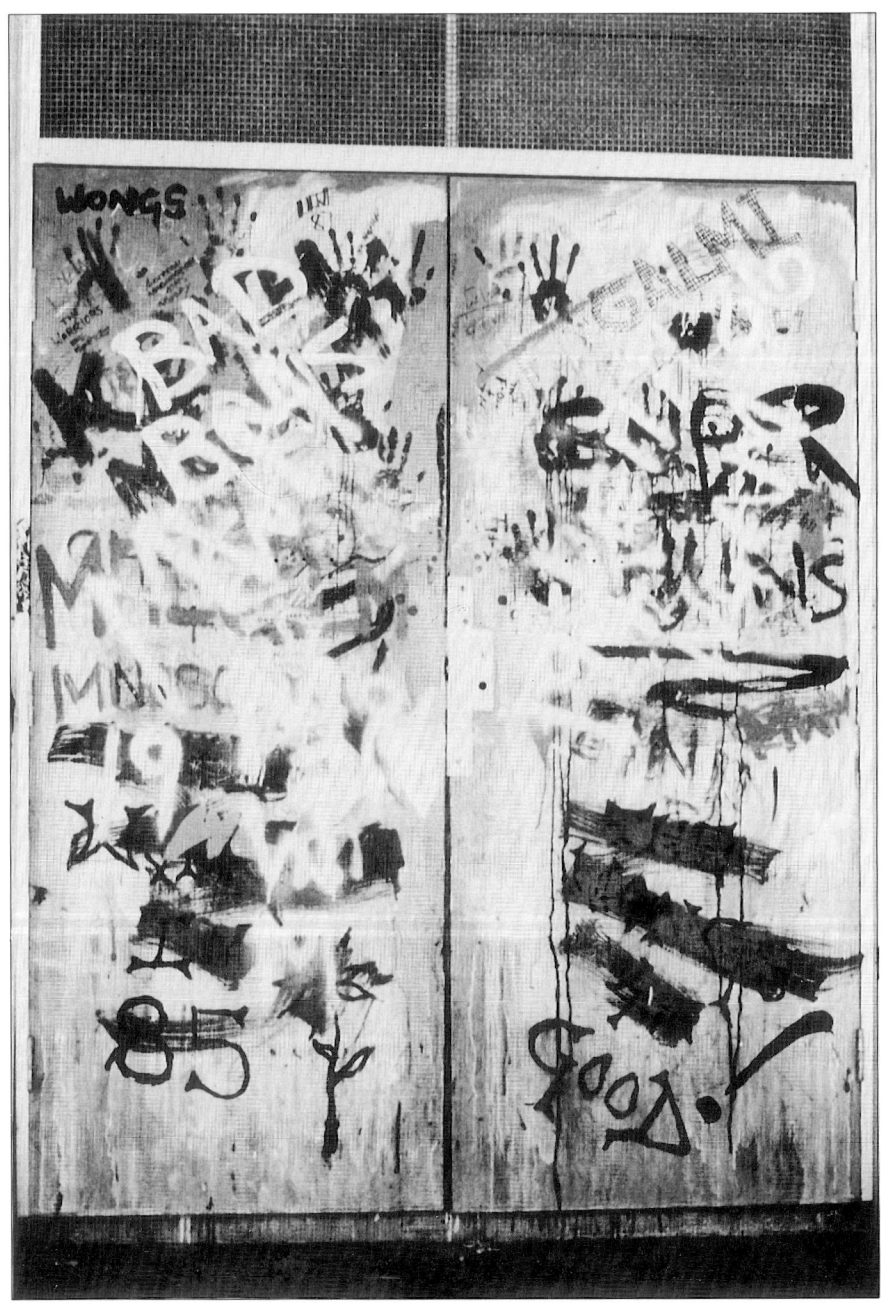

Plate 7: Graffiti on school doors in east Arnhem Land

bodies like paint, together with armbands, necklaces and long earrings. Battle fatigues (of the ex-army variety) are popular, especially heavy canvas lace-up boots in khaki, and military-style caps. Long trousers, either denim or camouflage, are *de rigueur* for these young men, in sharp contrast to men around them who, in the north, invariably wear shorts. The denims are tight, and often slashed deliberately, giving an impression of hard wear and tatters. Towels or T-shirts are often draped over the wearer's head, or tied on, giving the appearance of an Arab headdress. One man had a 'mohawk' haircut.

To complete this dramaturgy, the youth of these communities, and notably the petrol sniffers, listen to music and share the sound with all within earshot by blasting it out of large 'ghetto blaster' cassette players. The cassette players are invariably slung over one shoulder, speakers outward, so that all may hear the music. The music is hard rock and heavy metal.[15] The style of this music is in marked contrast to the rock played by local Aboriginal bands in the area (and throughout the Centre and the Territory),[16] the Christian-inspired pop music relayed at Aboriginal 'Fellowship' meetings, and the more relaxed country and western music favoured by older Aborigines. In east Arnhem Land on several occasions I witnessed deliberate attempts by groups of sniffers to drown out the communal Christian singing and amplified evangelical Cliff Richard songs with their clashing metal music.

In order to comprehend fully the degree of this oppositional youth culture, it is important to realise that these displays are taking place in some of the most tradition-oriented communities in Australia. While there have been changes, especially over the last two decades, in the degree of adherence to accepted practices, ritual and ceremonial life is strong, as are responsibilities and ties to country. Boys are initiated into the knowledge and ritual practices of Aboriginal Law, and ceremonies involving large numbers of people from the surrounding area are frequent. Rules governing desecration of sites and ceremonies are strictly enforced, to the extent that compensation is demanded from transgressors be they Aboriginal or non-Aboriginal. There are strict rules governing conduct between certain kin, particularly that of brothers and sisters towards each other. The placing of prohibitive taboos (known as 'cursing') on individuals, property and specific locations is a frequent occurrence. A man's curse can close the store or a section of shoreline (thus preventing fishing). A woman can curse her hands, preventing her from cooking, and parents might curse their daughter if they want to prevent her from marrying. This serious act places the cursed object or person in the sacred domain; it can only be counteracted by ritual intervention — by smoking out the cursed place and through the involvement of the individuals known as the *djunggayi* (managers) for particular ceremonies (see Burbank 1980).

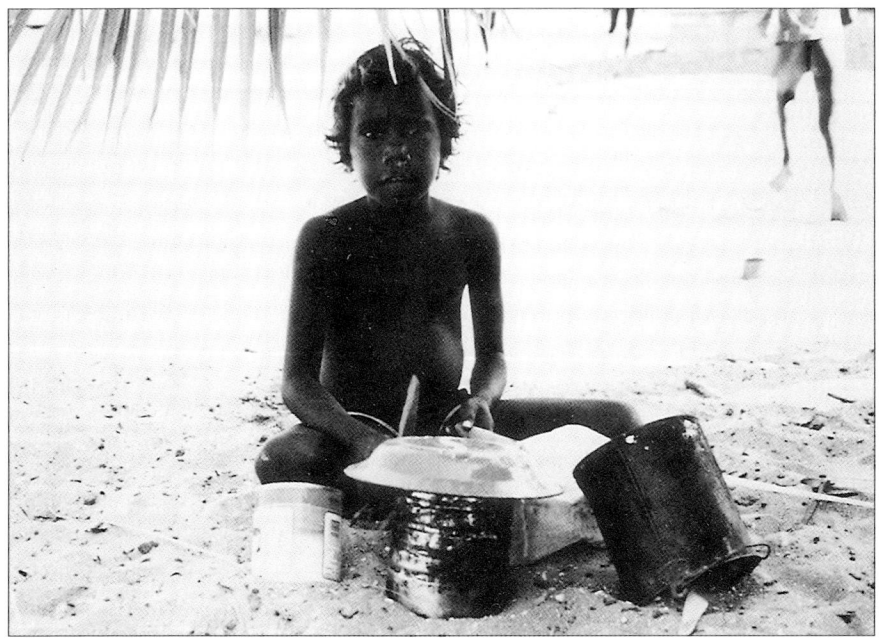

Plate 8: Rock musician in east Arnhem Land

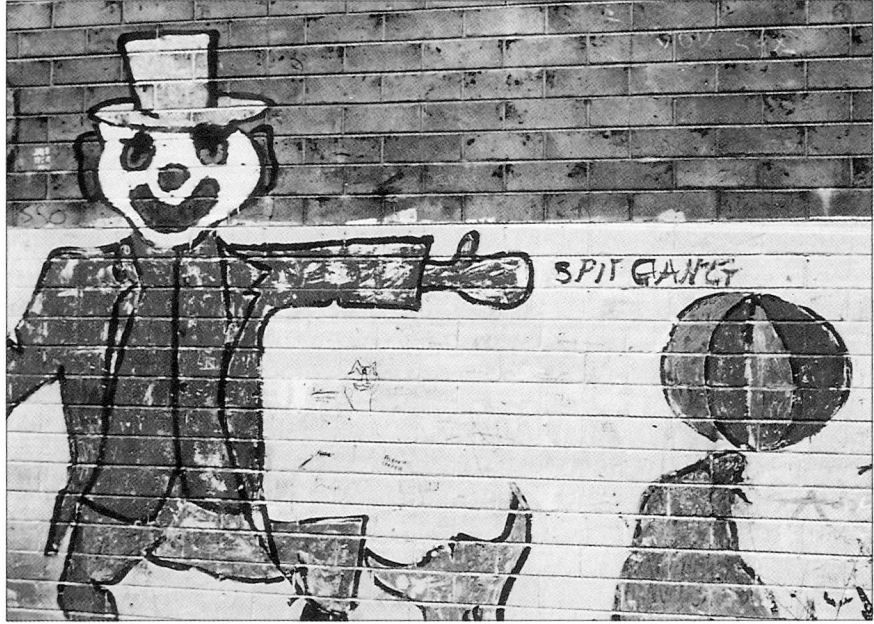

Plate 9: The Spit Gang leave their mark on a school mural, north-central Arnhem Land

Apart from the vigorous ceremonial life, there is also a strong Christian movement in these east Arnhem Land communities, an outcome of the presence of the Church Missionary Society of the Anglican Church, which established missions in the region from 1908 onwards. Three communities, Ngukurr (previously Roper River), Numbulwar and Angurugu, now have their own ordained Aboriginal ministers. Regular Bible Camps of a week's duration and nightly 'Fellowship' meetings are held in all three settlements. Baptisms and healing sessions, hymn singing and personal testimonials also occur. The region is also marked for its revival movements, which originated in a revival that occurred on Elcho Island in March 1979, and the development of a grassroots Aboriginal Christianity. There is inevitably some conflict arising from the strong role played by Christian movements in the midst of communities whose members vigorously pursue Aboriginal religious practices, but at least some people manage to participate successfully in both. A woman friend in one community devoted herself with equal energy to the annual Bible Camp, and to the preparations and dancing the following week for the circumcision of eight young boys. A spokesman at Nungalinya College (a theological college for Aboriginal people) in Darwin, himself a Fijian Christian, explained (S Renata, personal communication) that:

> The Aboriginal Ministers emphasise the whole man. They are free to use their own illustrations to help people understand. Before, they said traditional things were pagan; now they see it needs retaining. They try to encourage the Aboriginal people to retain the 'good' part of their ceremony — there is no perfect culture. R___ [Aboriginal Minister] has a free decision on his involvement with ceremony and little by little they help the people.

So it is against this backdrop of keen adherence to religious law — both Aboriginal and Christian — that the Warriors, the Wongs and the German Rebels, armed with their knives and their heavy metal music, the graffiti and petrol cans, present themselves. Such juvenile gangs have been interpreted by the sociologists studying deviance as having compensatory functions, in which subordinate groups formed gangs in their leisure time to develop alternative sources of self-esteem. In the gang, the core values of the straight world — sobriety, conformity and so on — were replaced by their opposites — hedonism, defiance of authority and the quest for kicks (Hebdige 1979, 76). The question of adolescents' perceptions of their own identity is also important. The struggle for definition of the 'self' is part of adolescence, and is 'made through rejection of, and rebellion against, those significant role models closest to the individual — one's parents and close members of the extended family' (Harris 1988, 7). Among Port Moresby Rascals, young men newly arrived in the city flee their negative identities (unemployed, worthless) and take on new names and identities. Harris (1988, 8) writes:

> Everywhere the intent is the same — to adopt a completely new, and preferably threatening or courageous identity. It is...designed to be noticed and to have impact. The young man wants to prove to himself that he can have an effect on the world around him...this is the rationale behind the resulting graffiti. The young man writes his name on every available space...he gives concrete, visible form to his new identity, thus assuring himself, as well as others, of his own reality.

The young Aborigines of east Arnhem Land are probably not subject to the same acute stresses experienced by Papua New Guineans who leave their villages for life in the city, but it is hard to ignore the fact that young Aborigines are consciously seeking alternatives to what their society has to offer. The style, the sounds and the actions which they adopt are spectacular symbols of non-acquiescence; a refusal of incorporation.

This discussion has focussed on the context of the maintenance or continuance of the drug use, rather than its commencement. My point is this: once the full array of oppositional styles has been sampled, as it were, by certain users of petrol, and has been found to offer a degree of subcultural cohesion, shared experiences and allure, this will offer a long-term outlet for those segments of the youth population attracted by risk and outrageousness. Within such a context, it is necessary for them to shrug off the entreaties of concerned adults, sympathetic white staff (some of whom are 'missionaries') and warnings of dangers to health. These entreaties could be seen to reinforce the heavy metal sniffers' chosen and self-conscious antipathy to the mainstream of respectable Aboriginal settlement life. In the terminology of the sociology of deviance, this is 'secondary deviance', reinforced and reinvented as a result of the labelling process. According to Cohen (1966, 24), to refer to individuals (as I, admittedly, and others do) as 'the sniffers' is to suggest

> someone who is normally or habitually given to certain kinds of deviance; who may be expected to behave in this way; who is literally a bundle of odious or sinister qualities. [The label] activates sentiments and calls out responses in others; rejection, contempt, suspicion, withdrawal, fear, hatred.

Once in this role, it is difficult (even if it is desired) for an individual to extricate him or herself from the group. One Council chairman, sincerely devoted to 'doing something' for the young people in terms of sport and recreation, told me, 'I'm fighting a war with these sniffers. I'll find something, and if they beat me, I'll keep trying. But they taunt the other kids, saying: "You're frightened of the Council, you're chicken".'

Significantly, it is marriage that brings about a cessation of sniffing for many male users — marriage is perceived to cause young men to 'settle down'. For young women, having a child is the precipitant for abstention. In a north-central Arnhem Land community where I had access to birth records, I found that female sniffers, for the most part, ceased using petrol when they bore a child. Eleven per cent of births (twenty-one) over a three-year period (1986–88) were to girls who had been sniffers. Of these twenty-one girls, only three were still using petrol after having borne a child. Others who gave up their sniffing had become Christians: they exchanged one social group and social status for another. By marrying, bearing a child or becoming a convinced Christian, the ex-sniffer discovers a new range of experiences and social responsibilities that serve to dislodge the focus on the drug use and its associated lifestyle.

REFUSING INCORPORATION

This chapter has explored a range of issues which arose out of my ethnography. There is a regional differentiation in this data, with the emphasis on sniffers-as-anorexics being located in Central Australian desert communities, and the subculture of gangs and the heavy metal style being found in Arnhem Land. Both these developments relate symbolically to notions of personal autonomy, to the body and resistance to 'bossing'. There is much that could be theorised about in these issues, and little opportunity to verify such theories. Nevertheless, one suggestion needs to be made about the latent and symbolic meaning of the behaviours I have witnessed and the comments I have collected, which relates primarily to young men in these Aboriginal communities. Young men and adolescent boys are evidently using petrol sniffing as an attempted solution to major crises of self-image and identity. Others have noted this before, suggesting that sniffing and gaol terms are contemporary 'initiation rites' for those experiencing social and cultural breakdown. Although there have been changes, in — and perhaps some losses of — social and religious practices in the regions I studied, the 'real' initiations are still in place, they have not been abandoned. But the crisis of identity still exists. The indicators for this lie in the rejection of identification with parents — with receiving food and being nurtured, with being 'fat' and healthy. 'I don't want to be like woman' was the phrase used by a teenage boy choosing to become thin and lean through sniffing. 'Mary Jane only. No men' was the announcement written on the T-shirt worn by a twenty-year-old woman in one desert community. She weighed only thirty-five kilograms. Control over one's own body is, in a sense, a last resort, the ultimate expression of influence over something. 'It's my own body! It's me sniffing' are statements of resistance and personal autonomy which have no political or social design, for the resistance is directed to those in the closest interpersonal realm. My interpretation of the resistance associated with sniffing thus differs substantially from that offered by Folds (1987) who raises it to a conscious political level.

The assumption by many observers that 'initiation' — the ritual processes that mark the passage from childhood to adulthood — magically produces a change of heart and an instant maturity is naive, for there is nothing automatic about adherence to customary rules or to societal expectations. Many users of petrol are socially and ritually 'men' rather than boys; both in the desert and in the north men in their twenties and occasionally those in their early thirties use petrol as a drug. Perhaps what is overlooked in the discussions about this ritualised transformation into an adult is that it constitutes an incorporation. While incorporation into the ranks of 'men' confers some rights and privileges, it also requires a sacrifice. I have described the wide freedoms of childhood in Aboriginal Australia, the absence of an authoritarian moulding of the child and the subsequent absence of a submissive attitude to adults: all these must be sacrificed by an individual becoming an adult. Hamilton (1981, 153) remarks:

> This is a pattern quite different from that encountered in most societies, including our own. For our children, the suppression of individual desires and submission to adult authority occurs at a very early age.... . The child's acceptance and sense of self-worth depends on it accepting the dictates of others, almost invariably its parents, who have absolute and unquestionable control even to the point of physical attack. By the time a child reaches puberty a high level of 'repression' has already taken place and adolescence becomes a struggle to rediscover and assert a long-surrendered autonomy. For the Aboriginal child, on the other hand, adolescence represents the first surrender.

By sniffing petrol and adopting the non-conformist style often associated with the practice, young people are refusing to surrender — or more specifically they are further delaying the inevitable embrace of mainstream life. Sniffing prolongs the period in which individual desires and autonomy can be expressed. For some, this process may become one-sided or unbalanced, as in the instances where the individual becomes pathologically self-absorbed in his or her body, because all other avenues of power are perceived to be curtailed. This absorption may eventually end in death. In other instances, personal autonomy takes a more 'rational' form of expression through identification with images of modernity such as clothing, rock music and graffiti, and through identification with social groupings intent upon impression-maintenance. Many of my informants argued that the young were neither unloved nor neglected, and perhaps it is time to deflect the focus in the analysis of Aboriginal drug use from a preoccupation with pathogenesis. Aboriginal society in these regions is not sick, but is engaged in a process of reworking itself and its values. The perceptions and concerns expressed by Aboriginal people that I have reproduced here say as much; perhaps we should take notice of them.

NOTES

1. Warner's use of the term Murngin to describe northeast Arnhem Land people is now superseded by the term Yolngu, used by those people to identify themselves as distinct from other groups.

2. That is 'think about' or take notice of.

3. Talk back (or 'back-answer') indicates answering back, or arguing. Another Aboriginal English expression used in this context is 'you make me talk', that is, 'you are forcing me to argue with you'.

4. Similar driving performances involving 'doing wheelies' and kicking up dust accompanied by squealing brakes have become a modern way of demonstrating anger and going 'berserk' for both sober and inebriated individuals. It always provokes a strong audience response.

5. In Western Australian desert communities sniffers use this term for petrol. In Arnhem Land, the argot of sniffers refers to 'fuel'.

6. 'Too much' means ample, plenty.

7. I am grateful to Marika Moisseef for drawing these references to my attention.

8. It is likely that missionaries (both in the Centre and the Top End) promoted milk as a healthy drink. At Ngukurr the Anglican mission kept goats which were cared for by Aboriginal children (now adults) for their milk. Regular milk was issued by the Mission School at Ngukurr in the 1950s (Church Missionary Society 1953). Aboriginal Health Workers at Ngukurr reported that they administer milk as an antidote to poisoning. On one occasion a boy swallowed engine oil and on another a child ingested some medication by mistake: both were made to drink large quantities of milk.

9. Sibthorpe 1988, 351.

10. The first Aboriginal men to be offered English wine — by Captain Cook's landing party in January 1788 — promptly spat it out (Hughes 1988, 85).

11. *Ngurpa* can mean: 1. unfamiliar, inexperienced; 2. not competent, unable to do something; 3. not knowing a fact or person; 4. being an abstainer (of cigarettes, liquor etc) (Goddard 1987, 84).

12. PS means petrol sniffer.

13 Harris (1988) documents the evolution of Rascal gangs in Papua New Guinea from disorganised juvenile groups to disciplined and sometimes violent criminal gangs. Gangs included the Four Mile Rascals, Raipex, Harlem Lords, Tigers, Rough Riders, Devils and KKK (1988, 43). In the Caribbean, collective movements of disenchanted youth were called 'rude-boys' and 'warriors' (Mahabir 1988).

14. Adults interpret these to be 'just pretending — like wearing necklace', or else 'from fights'.

15. The international heavy metal rock bands have names such as Megadeath, Slayer and Poison (see also Hebdige 1979, 155).

16. At an Aboriginal Rock Music Festival in Darwin in September 1988, over twenty Aboriginal bands performed. Many record and distribute their own songs through Aboriginal media organisations.

CHAPTER

SANCTIONS

In recent years, anthropological and social analyses of drug use have tended to stress the role played by social learning and ritual in the creation of culturally established restraints that serve to limit human drug use. Ritual, in this context, refers to the stylised behaviours in which drug users administer the drug, select the setting for use, engage in activities after the drug ingestion and create methods of preventing untoward effects (Harding and Zinberg 1977, 12; Pearson 1987; Lindstrom 1987). Apart from these acquired interpersonal restraints, regulation of drug use may be formal and legislative in nature, as in prohibition. There may also be unequal rights to consume a substance which serve to restrict its use on the grounds of gender identity, distinctions between young and old, pagan and Christian, modern and traditional, sane and insane, knowledgeable and ignorant. All these cultural demarcations serve as restraints on drug use (see Lindstrom 1987). These researchers describe how the interaction of set and setting variables can provide an environment in which self-regulation is practised by drug users: alcohol users decide they have 'had enough'; marijuana users pause after smoking to determine their level of mood-change; those taking psychedelic drugs carefully stage-manage their environment, their companions, and ensure they have an experienced user present (Zinberg 1984; Pearson 1987).

In the previous chapter, I have described the social learning and some of the rituals associated with petrol sniffing: the induction of new users, the settings for use and the creative style of using groups. I have also touched upon some of the distinctions which exist: sniffing is the preoccupation of adolescents and young adults rather than the mature-aged; of boys more so than girls; of the decidedly non-Christian and the modern; and of those deemed 'knowledgeable' rather than 'ignorant' of the use of the substance. However, it appears that, at the present stage of this drug use among Aborigines, these contextual restraints have been insufficient to prevent untoward sequelae associated with overuse: chronic social disorder; acute physical and psychological symptoms; repeated hospitalisation and, in some cases, death. Although many users select methods of administering the substance which may minimise harm, for example, sniffing in the open air, using small containers and sniffing in public places, others sniff petrol continuously or as often as possible, using large tins, and engage in dangerous activities such as climbing roofs, lighting fires or swimming out to sea. In one socio-cultural group, a few determined users were literally sniffing themselves to death by deliberately losing weight. Apart from those individuals who decide to give up sniffing for a variety of reasons, I have no evidence that using groups have yet developed effective group restraints that would assist moderation.

Pamela Watson (1987, 119–20) reported:

> In the early 1960s biomedical scientists investigating drug-seeking behaviour produced evidence indicating that moderate drug use is not a natural phenomena [sic]. Instead, it occurs as a result of socio-cultural controls imposed upon what now appears to be the 'normal' situation — that is, open-ended use unrestrained by appetite or satiation...Drugs are experienced as inherently rewarding *in a situation free of negative social sanction*. This results in repetition of the actions which lead to the consumption of the drug in the first instance, and thus to continuous use.

Her suggestion that moderation only occurs as a result of imposed socio-cultural controls is alarming and salutary, for it is clear that many users of petrol as an inhalant have not yet perceived the need for restraint. This may be because Aboriginal evaluations of sensual activities (as in some other societies) mean that whether one is eating, drinking, smoking — or sniffing petrol — then it should be done until the effects are felt as fully as possible (Strathern 1987, 237). In addition, the level of tolerance and acceptance of the practice of sniffing among some populations has enabled this situation to persist.

The situation in Aboriginal communities where sniffing is practised by a proportion of the youthful population is not, however, always one in which 'anything goes'. Although it has taken time, in some cases, for social opinion to become mobilised towards the creation of negative sanctions, these are now increasingly apparent. This chapter discusses some formal and informal sanctions in place, as well as addressing frankly some of the impediments to their successful operation.

INFORMAL LOCAL SANCTIONS

Informal and locally based sanctions underway in communities include both punitive and diversionary interventions formulated by the local community, sometimes in conjunction with outside assistance. Some communities have appointed a 'warden', a male Aboriginal community member, equipped sometimes with a motorbike, whose role is to patrol the community dissuading sniffers from sniffing. This is usually accomplished by confronting users and pouring out their petrol supplies, breaking up using groups and urging youngsters to return to their houses or camps. It rarely involves physical punishment as this can bring an angry response from the youth's relatives. In other cases, sniffers have received formal physical punishment at the hands of councillors or parents under Council auspices.

Such occasions are usually public affairs, staged so that individuals experience the double effects of physical pain and psychological discomfort associated with being made to feel shame in the eyes of witnesses. Physical punishment of this order appears to be more common in the north than in Central Australian communities, and had only been deemed successful in two settlements I visited. Sniffers have been locked up on occasions in impromptu 'gaols' in settlements, usually as a last resort by councillors or wardens. Some coastal settlements have sent petrol sniffers away, in a form of temporary exile, to islands where they have been forced to hunt and fish for survival. Others have been taken to outstations or bush camps away from their home township, where attempts have been made to engage their interest in hunting or fishing, fence building, camel catching and other activities.

Diversionary recreational schemes, sometimes simply the provision of a building equipped with darts, a pool table and weightlifting equipment, are frequently mooted by Aborigines and non-Aboriginal advisors, in attempts to deflect the attention and interests of the sniffing groups. Sport is often perceived to be a solution to juvenile restlessness and a highly effective method of raising self-esteem. Boxing, for example, is promoted as a sport in which the competitors can rely only on themselves rather than 'hiding behind the team' (Mason and Wilson 1988, 105). An overview of the successes and failures of these interventions is provided by Morice et al (1981). More relevant to this discussion are the responses of Aboriginal people to some of these endeavours — responses which have not always been supportive — and in order to analyse this, an understanding of the cultural context is helpful. First, some vignettes derived from fieldwork observations.

> In a desert community, the fathers and grandfathers of petrol sniffers take up spears and other weapons to accost the community-appointed 'wardens' whose job it is to rebuke sniffers and pour away their petrol.
>
> A man takes an axe to break open the lock of a makeshift 'gaol' in his community where sniffers had been restrained after a particularly wild rampage. He did so to release his own son, a chronic sniffer.
>
> A couple who received government assistance in the form of a Toyota to run a camp for petrol sniffers finally gave up the enterprise after jealous accusations from other community members that they would not share the use of the vehicle.
>
> A series of communities received a grant of $5,000 each to be spent on some resources or activities to benefit young people and divert petrol sniffers. One community purchased several dozen pairs of roller

skates so that youngsters could skate in the community hall. Another bought swings and playground equipment. A third complemented the grant with other funds and purchased a four-wheel drive vehicle, ostensibly to take the sniffers out bush — it was taken over by one family, then stolen and wrecked. A fourth community used the money to repair a vehicle for use by the young people — the vehicle was never used in the manner intended. In another community the white community adviser purchased lawn mowers.

'At a Christian Fellowship meeting [Arnhem Land], two boys walked through the service sniffing petrol. A man (Z) took the petrol from them, threw it out and gave them a smack. They went and told X and he came to the service with a bundle of spears. He was taking partner for his [son's child]. He threw one. It is a good thing Y was there, he stopped that old man. This morning X didn't eat any breakfast, he just picked up a boomerang and started arguing. [Those two boys] did this because they were angry that Z smacked them. They didn't like him telling them not to sniff.' (Burbank, personal communication)[1]

These incidents touch upon a series of themes which mark the very core of the 'problem' with petrol sniffing. The themes are common throughout the different regions studied and relate on the one hand to matters 'cultural', and on the other to access to resources and interactions with bureaucracy. They are the issues avoided by the bland assertions that Aboriginal communities should take responsibility for actions and interventions associated with petrol sniffing, and those which most frustrate the front-line field officers and government representatives who must implement government policies.

SOCIO-CULTURAL INFLUENCES

Primary among the socio-cultural contexts that affect local attempts at intervention are the themes of individual autonomy, interpersonal loyalties and the behaviour expected of kin. The pre-eminence of the value attributed to individual autonomy has been touched upon earlier. This high value placed upon an individual's rights not to be 'bossed' by others, together with the acceptance of expressions of independence by young people, coexist, contrarily, within a society marked by elaborate rules of conduct and a high level of conformity. This is illustrated aptly by Harris (1984, 38):

> M___ a Yolngu carpenter of about twenty-five years of age, had fixed the cabin on his family's twenty-foot boat. But all his brothers kept sitting on top of it and broke it again. He started

to repair it the second time and put stronger timber in the frame, and he said, 'They always sit on it'. And I said, 'Can't you explain that it will break if they do?' And he said, 'No, they won't take any notice. We can't tell each other things like that'. The brothers would express their independence by sitting on the cabin roof, but the carpenter brother could not aggressively express his own individuality by adopting a leadership role.

In the normal course of events people are able to balance these values, so that autonomy and restraint are enacted in appropriate circumstances. A variety of subtle techniques are brought to bear which enable people to negotiate difficult situations. For example, when a middle-aged man told how he had given up drinking alcohol, he said he used to leave his money at home and only take $2 with him to the pub, so that when people asked him for money he could truthfully say he had none. 'But if someone asks for food here [in his home settlement] and I say no, that's shame to me, make me feel ashamed. If I've got only one packet of tea, I've got to give it. But if I give too much, my own family go hungry.'

The role and composition of the family are frequently said to be factors that affect the prevalence of petrol sniffing, and several interventions (and many reported theories of the aetiology of sniffing) are based upon the premise that family dysfunction or social breakdown are responsible for the psychological and social despair which are thought to precipitate sniffing. Rather than attempting to prove or disprove this hypothesis, it is important to provide some analysis of the perfectly healthy, socially acceptable and firmly 'traditional' ways of doing things which have, as unfortunate side effects, undermined initiatives by Aboriginal people themselves.

Aboriginal populations in the regions covered by the study support each other primarily through the immediate family. It is not so long ago that, among some Western desert groups for example, the available network of individuals living together totalled only eight or twelve family members (Peterson and Long 1986), with the nearest neighbours being within a day's walk, perhaps thirty kilometres. This placed a high premium on family solidarity. Today, despite high levels of mutual cooperation on a large scale (for example, during ceremonial periods), Aboriginal 'communities' still operate as a series of family groups with a minimal level of large group cohesion in some cases. Even if an Aboriginal settlement is composed of people united by a common language and by shared rights to land (certainly not always the case), the population can still be riven by dissent between opposed family groups and individuals. Both Fred Myers (writing of Central Australia) and Nancy Williams (writing of Arnhem Land) have noted the absence of a concept of 'community welfare', an absence which can give the social environment an egocentric quality (Myers 1986; Williams 1987). Williams also questions the common assertion that in small face-to-face societies individual rights are sacrificed in order to maintain 'social harmony' or 'group survival': she emphasises the individual quality of disputes and their settlement. Incidents involving the kin of petrol sniffers, who act to defend them against dispute or punishment, are notable for the degree of self-help involved. They do not generally go before a 'jural public' for adjudication by the consensus of the community. This is not the occasion to enter into a prolonged discussion on Aboriginal disputation and leadership, but a brief mention is called for, as notions of responsibility, authority and social controls necessarily touch upon the dilemma of dealing with sniffers at a local level.

Much has been written about the social controls thought to be implicit in Aboriginal customary Law and one of the most accurate and straightforward accounts is provided by Maddock (1984). First, he brings together the threads of the anthropological debate about the role of elders or Law men, with a quote from Hiatt (1965, 145–46):

> Old men had considerable prestige, especially in matters of religion, but they did not stand out as general leaders.... . Different persons therefore acted as organisers [of ceremonies etc] at different times, and there was nobody with permanent authority. Men of high ritual status played no special part in settling disputes.

Second, he makes a useful distinction between the committal of a public wrong and committal of a private wrong. Breaches of public binding norms (usually associated with religious Law) are most likely to be met with sanctions from those obliged to instigate them. However, breaches of private norms, resulting in quarrels or disputes, seldom involve an obvious clash between right and wrong. Maddock sees these as being breaches of non-binding norms, and they are no-one's particular 'business' to pass judgment on or to intervene. However, if such private disputes entail violent disturbances, then bystanders and others may try to stop them before they go too far (Maddock 1984, 230). Such intervention is not obligatory for anyone in particular, but constitutes an 'anonymous collective' action to restore peace. These comments provide further evidence of the autonomy of the individual. Those involved in a dispute may resort to verbal or physical self-help producing

> acceptable but opposed arguments (for example insistence on a right, accusation of meanness)...occasionally a person would defy 'the code of good conduct' and ride roughshod over 'the legitimate interests of others' — and still emerge the winner.

This helps to explain, in part, why a father who attacks a petrol-sniffing warden can argue that his actions are justified. He is not necessarily obligated by fatherly duty to remonstrate with a warden who interferes with his son's actions (although there are strong societal reasons why he should so take issue). Not every man in the same circumstances would take similar action, nevertheless a man could justify doing so. In terms of the 'non-binding norm' that no outside person has the right to deal with his son in such a manner, he rightfully and justifiably resorts to self-help. The warden is equally in a position to argue that the community has placed upon him the responsibility to intervene if he encounters petrol sniffing. This is not, then, a matter of Aboriginal Law (the father's actions) versus 'white instigated rules' (the warden's actions) but a matter of negotiation between flexible sets of norms. A man or woman does not always take kindly to others passing judgment on that individual nor on members of his or her close kin. Women are quick to deny that their husbands drink alcohol or that their son sniffs petrol. Questioning by an outsider about such issues is likely to produce acute embarrassment.

The most fundamental reason why close kin maintain at least an outward expression of solidarity is that kin and self are, on one level, indistinguishable. This is illustrated by the linguistic terms used. In several Western Desert languages, for example, the term *walytja* specifies a sense of relatedness meaning 'kin' and 'family'. In Pintupi, it is used to refer not only to one's own possessions but also to oneself (Myers 1986, 109). One's kin are conceptually part of one's self and those referred to as *walytja* have a shared identity with the speaker. This shared identity also links humankind with the land, so that among Pitjantjatjara speakers, for example, certain others are referred to as *ngurawalytja*, which means literally 'country relations' — people who are kin because they share ownership and rights in the land, who are actually related to the land. Among the Pintupi, a person is believed to be made up of maternal blood and paternal bone (Myers 1986, 105), which provides a further insight into the way in which people conceptualise their close family. Pitjantjatjara people divide themselves into one of two moieties which group together members of alternate generation levels. So a person distinguishes himself, his siblings and cousins as one generation level moiety, and his parents and their siblings and so on in another — the two moieties are referred to as *nganantarka* (our bones) and *tjanamiltjan* (their flesh). European Australians have a similar conceptual framework when they refer to 'our own flesh and blood'. Nunggubuyu speakers in east Arnhem Land say that a father gives a child his face and his feet, where a footprint is as individual as a face (Burbank 1980, 33). With an understanding of these concepts which underlie relationships between kin, it is possible to appreciate the reasons why an assault (even a metaphorical one) upon a son is tantamount to an assault upon his father.

When a social worker interviews parents about the sniffing activities of their child, the integrity of the parents is impugned because they and the child have a shared identity. An angry or defensive response may be expressed, not because the parents condone the activities of a petrol-sniffing child (although they may tacitly do so), but because the shared understandings that make up kinship and relatedness require them to enact the ideal — support for kin. They must officially represent themselves as 'speaking up' for their child. In private, of course, close kin may express quite different views. 'Speaking up' or 'taking part' are expressions used by Aboriginal people to describe these obligatory public interventions. In different regions each socio-linguistic group has a variety of rules about who should support whom in disputes and fights. Burbank (1980, 66), for example, notes that at Numbulwar, east Arnhem Land, the following family members are expected to participate in each other's fights if participation is called for: mother/mother's brother:woman's child — father/father's sister:man's child — brother:brother — sister:sister. Mothers may either restrain or assist their children in a fight. Burbank also points out that these public disputes are not an example of cultural disintegration or the breakdown of law and order, but are examples of highly structured activity governed by cultural rules.

During one of my fieldwork visits to east Arnhem Land, the community Council staged a public beating of some young men who had been sniffing petrol. Although this had the tacit (and rather unwilling) approval of others, some women complained to me afterwards that it had not been right because some of those punished had been hit on the head. According to the 'rules' of physical altercation, the soft body parts and head are off-limits: 'You can hit them anywhere, arm, leg, rump, but not the head, that's *gudugudu* [forbidden]' (Burbank 1980, 69). In fact it was unlikely that their heads had been hit; by claiming a contravention of these rules, the women expressed their disapproval of the whole exercise. Since that time (1984), such direct punishment has been abandoned in this community. The chairman said that

> Council members don't like to get involved with parents' business, so the only way [with the sniffers] is to get sport and recreation going. If they sniff around town, any Council member has *no* right to punish them. There is no point, if the parents won't do anything [themselves].

Another Council member said bluntly 'If I give a hiding to a kid, his family come with spears'. The problem in these situations is that no-one takes consistent direct action to serve as a negative sanction. A young married man at the same community (who has a younger brother who is a chronic sniffer) told me 'Well, if I see sniffers, I don't do anything. That's for mother and father to do.'

Another reason why interventions of the type discussed (wardens, beatings) are often problematic is associated with shame. Shame is defined by Myers (1986, 120) to be 'usually associated with the discomfort of being observed by others in the public domain, especially at being seen to do something that is poor etiquette, ill-mannered or wrong'. Another anthropologist, Epstein (1984, 33), explained:

> It is...a response activated by an awareness or feeling that one's inadequacies have been or are about to be uncovered... . As Sartre...has eloquently expressed it: 'Shame is by nature recognition. I recognise that I am as the Other sees me.'

Ironically, the notion of shame, usually understood by anthropologists to be an important tool of social control (see Myers 1986; Epstein 1984), can serve the function of assisting petrol sniffers to maintain their use — in effect acting to undermine social controls. Why it is that shaming has not been used effectively to curb the activities of petrol sniffers is hard to say. Perhaps it is because once a group of sniffers of a 'critical mass' is established, the users are able to construct enough solidarity and adherence to their own in-group mores to withstand the pressure to feel shame about their pursuit. One of these mores is 'not to take notice of anybody', as several informants explained. If an individual is 'proud' of himself (as is said of some sniffers) and his actions, it is unlikely that shaming will be effective; it is only influential if a sense of inadequacy or of being found out is elicited. So only the parents and kin feel shame when someone else publicly remonstrates with their son or relative, not the subject of remonstration him or herself.

Children are commonly said to have no shame, because their maturity is not yet sufficient for them to experience embarrassment over their actions. However, a socialisation practice is to use the rebuke 'No shame!' when children engage in disapproved actions. Despite the fact that children rarely take any obvious notice of this purely verbal form of social control, ultimately they absorb the concept. The significant element in this discussion covering family loyalty and reactions to outside interference is that shame helps to separate what is defined as 'public' from what is defined as 'private'. A warden who confronts a petrol sniffer or who locks up another man's son is, from this perspective, flying in the face of acceptable practice. He may cause embarrassment to an isolated sniffer (without his peers) by publicly chastising him, but instead of this being allowed to take effect as a form of social control, an older kinsman, a father or grandfather steps in because he too is embarrassed and ashamed. Strictly speaking, the warden should also feel awkward (and many do) about being the instrument by which shame is inflicted on another. For this reason, Aboriginal people who become police aides, or who take upon themselves official social control positions, are forced to legitimise their role and metaphorically separate themselves by displaying markers of their distinct status (uniforms and official vehicles).

A variety of commentators on the supposed causes of petrol sniffing in some Aboriginal societies point to the lack of social cohesion as a result of the coexistence of several different language groups in one community. While there may be some truth in this, it is more likely that the disparate nature of a multi-language group may result in that community experiencing more difficulties in mustering a cohesive response to the practice, as a result of excessively complex politics within its population. However, even close-knit communities, linked by language, land holding and kinship associations, also encounter practical problems in acting against the practice. In order to illustrate this, let us examine the situation in some Western Desert communities using data derived from my research. In these examples I have disguised the names of the communities involved.

The total Aboriginal population of this region of Western Australia is just under 1,000 people, who live in seven settlements and a variety of outstations. Mobility is high, with frequent movement east into South Australia and west into the Goldfields region of Western Australia. Residents are linked by their shared socio-cultural and historical background, by religious practices and language — two major and very similar languages are used. The population of the region has arranged itself among the seven locations very much according to the desires of the residents themselves. A core group of the older generation was previously housed in a mission at The Hills until the mid-1970s, when the outstation movement enabled them to split up and reside on or close to their own lands. In other words, the residents of the outstations — which have now become settlements — are gathered there of their own free choice, with certain others who either share rights in that land, or have affinal links with landholders. The residents, then, share many elements which closely bind them to one another. There are also inter-settlement ties as a result of marriage. As examples we can take Whitesand and Blacksand communities.

The genealogy in Figure 10 shows the links between the G____ family (normally resident at Whitesand) and the M____ family (normally resident at Blacksand) — two locations which are geographically close. Blacksand has a persistent petrol-sniffing problem, while Whitesand has very few resident sniffers. As a result of the death of a family member, the M____ family core group (Mr M____ and his two wives, several of their children, sons or daughters-in-law, and grandchildren) moved to Whitesand to live for approximately six months. The death which prompted the move was that of Mr M____'s brother's son, and was caused

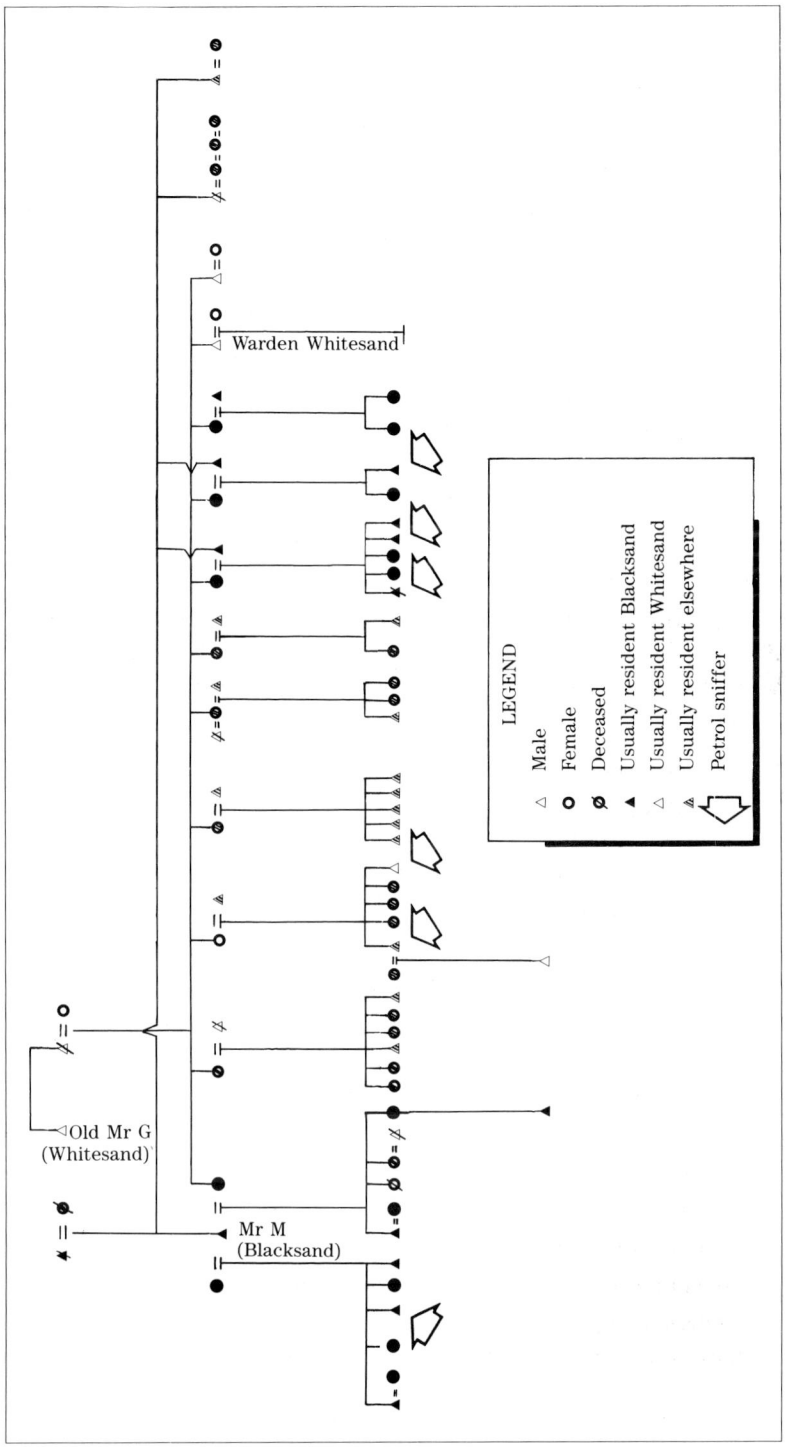

Figure 10: Genealogy of the G____ family (Whitesand) and the M____ family (Blacksand)

by petrol sniffing. While at Whitesand during their temporary residence, Mr M____'s own son (aged seventeen) persistently sniffed petrol, and three of Mr M____'s other nephews (sons of his second wife's sisters) who are also habitual users. The residents of Whitesand find it difficult to deal with the sniffing activities which surround Mr M____'s son, despite the fact that he is a 'visitor'. These difficulties arise because Mr M____'s two wives both come from Whitesand and they have many close relatives there. His second wife is, in fact, the daughter of old Mr G____, the man recognised locally as the senior traditional owner of the land upon which the settlement is built. Significantly, the Whitesand community has made old Mr G____'s son the community petrol-sniffing warden. The G____ family then, despite being residents of Whitesand, and concerned to keep their community free from the trouble associated with petrol sniffing, take no direct action against Mr M____ and his son. The other members of Whitesand cannot act either, because they would be taking action against the 'grandson' of the senior man of their own community.

The other notable feature linking the G____ family and the M____ family is the fact that three men of the M____ family, all brothers, are married to three women of the G____ family, all sisters. These ties bind the two communities of Whitesand and Blacksand even closer together. Furthermore, the remaining marriage and residential associations of the two families reach as far as Fregon (east, in the Pitjantjatjara Lands), and Laverton (west, in the Goldfields), with a scattering of kin in each of four local communities. The case of the M____ family and the G____ family occurs many times throughout the region and this closeness, together with the frequency of movement between communities, means that individuals who may be users of petrol may move freely between centres. Although at community meetings people make statements about 'keeping those sniffers out' (ie outside their community), in reality because all are related, there is no question of preventing their arrival nor of demanding their departure. The interesting aspect of this, from an outsider's point of view, is that nobody actually articulates this to be the nub of the problem (at least, not in public forums like meetings). There are expressions of irritation and sorrow that the young people persist in these activities, and exhortations that the 'community' should 'support' the Council. But no-one says 'Well, we really have a problem here because we are all so closely related that nobody wants to confront young Johnny there'; or 'How can we kick these three brothers out of our community when they are sons of that old man who is like a cousin for us?' This underlying explanation (or one of them) for the absence of firmness with petrol sniffers, is only apparent once the nature of the associations between people becomes clear.

The same problem afflicts community councils. At Blacksand, for example, which has around twenty resident sniffers, there is an Aboriginal Council made up of sixteen individuals. Of these, six (including the vice-chairman, and the warden) are in fact the parents of seven of the community's petrol sniffers. How, then, can the Council take a firm stance on petrol sniffing? Nevertheless the Council will (to varying degrees) meet with visiting teams from welfare or government agencies, and talk seriously about the petrol-sniffing problem without ever saying frankly that they are in a double bind, that they are confused, ashamed and embarrassed because their own children are also involved. The average age of a councillor at Blacksand is thirty-eight years, and the majority lived at The Hills, where they were born into a mission environment. A thirty-eight-year-old adult would have spent his first eight years in the mission-run dormitory (which closed in 1958) largely separated from his parents, and would have been fed and clothed throughout his young life by the mission, later the welfare authorities. Provision of meals and clothing for Aborigines at The Hills did not cease until 1978. If he misbehaved the missionaries gave him a hiding. By the age of twenty such an individual probably first encountered petrol sniffing, even participated in sniffing (ie in 1970, when it was first noted here), and now this thirty-eight-year-old has a thirteen-year-old son who habitually sniffs petrol.

While it is often asserted, and indeed has become a conventional wisdom, that petrol sniffing continues to be practised because previously tradition-oriented Aboriginal groups are 'losing' their culture and suffering from family 'breakdown', on the contrary it appears that in many instances traditional cultural mores are alive and well. People are behaving in an entirely appropriate manner in which they adhere to customary modes of conduct and family loyalties.

ACCESS TO RESOURCES

Competition for government resources is intense in many Aboriginal groups, particularly as the political climate of the Whitlam era has become muted by the economic realities of the 1980s and 1990s. The homelands (outstation) movement, despite philosophical and financial commitment from the federal government, is still the locus of federal–state friction over the provision of essential services. While not entirely devolving its responsibilities for outstation support upon the states, the federal government takes the view that general community services should be provided by state and territory governments (Commonwealth of Australia 1987, 100). The state and territory governments vary considerably in their allocations — the South Australian government provided no essential services funding, while the Northern Territory government provided $15.9 million between 1983 and 1986. The Queensland government provides no assistance at all to Aboriginal people who 'choose to move from established settlements' (Commonwealth of Australia 1987, 98).

In short, the homelands movement is alive and vigorous, but resources are sought competitively and funding is more likely to decline than it is to increase. The struggle to establish and maintain outstations is just one example in an arena of competition between Aboriginal groups for government assistance of varying kinds. This is what Gerritsen has termed the 'politics of scarcity' (Gerritsen 1982, 68). It is a particularly apt illustration in this instance, for outstations are often mooted as viable solutions to petrol sniffing. The evidence to support the suggestion that sniffing is less prevalent among outstation groups is quite strong. Maningrida, for example, has been subject to petrol sniffing for twenty years, while the practice is reported at only one of its more than thirty outstations, with a total population of over 500 permanent residents (Commonwealth of Australia 1987, 77-78). Oak Valley, the homeland centre established out of Yalata, South Australia, is another example. Yalata had a fluctuating incidence of petrol sniffing between 1976 and 1989, while the homeland community (which exchanges residents constantly with Yalata) had none. However, some locations which began their existence as outstations have developed into settlements and now have petrol sniffing in their midst. This is the case with several Pitjantjatjara and Ngaanyatjarra locations in south and western Australia.

Apart from the suggestion that life on outstations in itself tends to deter users of petrol from sniffing (or else does not attract chronic users who prefer settlement life), some outstations have attempted to function specifically as rehabilitation centres for sniffers (Coombs et al 1983, 320-35). Some of these attempts have come to grief as a result of power struggles among key individuals and families and because of disputes arising out of selective government assistance. These incidents tend to reinforce Gerritsen's suggestion that the establishment of outstations enables enterprising individuals to create and maintain a power base by authoritatively attracting government support (Gerritsen 1982), rather than simply satisfying spiritual needs (Japanangka and Nathan 1983). In an environment where outstations and vehicles are both highly valued resources, their variable distribution among Aboriginal populations is bound to cause friction at times. Vehicles are particularly problematic, being expensive (a Toyota Landcruiser now costs approximately $35,000) and easily damaged and their use is subject to intense local politicking. Toyotas are the resource par excellence requested by Aboriginal people in remote communities. In 1984 the Aboriginal Benefits Trust Account, which receives royalties under the Aboriginal Land Rights (Northern Territory) Act 1976, devoted 46 per cent ($2 million) of its grant moneys to vehicle purchases.

Many 'community'-instigated programs to curb petrol sniffing request a vehicle as part of the program, either to take sniffers out bush or to assist in the mobility of local field officers. Local frictions can be exacerbated in such instances and eventually bring about the demise of these so-called interventions. Frictions usually arise for two main reasons: the scarcity of resources and competing claims for control of, and access to, the vehicle. In the midst of these competing interests, the altruistic reasons for requesting the vehicle in the first place (to do something constructive to divert petrol sniffers) sometimes become lost. Awareness of these issues is an essential prerequisite for funding allocations aimed at sniffing programs. The State Working Party on Petrol Sniffing (Western Australia) consistently resisted numerous requests for vehicles for these reasons. There are usually available vehicles which are 'community-owned' which could, if desired, be used for sniffer-related projects. But as one community adviser observed, when space on a vehicle is at a premium, the dogs get thrown off first and then the children in order to make room for an adult who wishes to go out. The children can often be left to their own devices for the day.

In this discussion, I have shown that there are aspects of Aboriginal social life and perceptions which profoundly influence the way in which people think about, and deal with, petrol sniffing. On the surface, some of the instances described appear to show that Aboriginal people are unconcerned about the practice. Among some segments of populations this may well be true; petrol sniffing among the kin of other people is not their concern because it is not their business. Others, involved on a day-to-day basis with the issue, have been forced to accommodate it in a variety of ways. Some attempts at decisive action have been impeded, ironically, by strongly operating cultural factors emphasising personal autonomy and family loyalty. The problem of access to government resources has also exacerbated intra-community friction, contributing to the demise of some attempts at intervention in petrol sniffing.

THE ROLE OF CHRISTIANITY

In both of the regions in which my research was focussed — east Arnhem Land and the Western Desert — there have been Aboriginal-inspired Christian revivals in the 1980s. In addition, both regions have a history of the involvement of larger Christian missionary enterprises. Although both forms of Christianity fluctuate in popularity and commitment over time, Aboriginal Christians now form significant groups. As such they have also influenced attitudes towards petrol sniffing. In east Arnhem Land particularly, the Christian movement has devoted considerable attention to petrol sniffing, so constituting yet another influence on sniffers — another setting variable which serves to exert control over, and express disapproval of, their behaviour.

FROM ANGLICANS TO ACTION

The three east Arnhem Land settlements of Ngukurr, Angurugu and Numbulwar were established by the Church Missionary Society (CMS) of the Anglican Church in 1908, 1921 and 1952 respectively. Although all are now incorporated communities no longer officially designated as 'missions', the Anglican Church maintains strong links with the settlements, providing linguists (several with years of experience in local languages and Bible translation), assisting at major events such as Bible Camps, and having ordained three Aboriginal ministers, one in each location. Naturally, the Christians espouse temperance, preach against alcoholic beverages and petrol sniffing and disapprove of smoking. Indeed, in the 1940s, the CMS missions in which the adults of today were raised refused to distribute the government tobacco ration on the grounds that it was an addictive substance (Cole 1980, 66). In 1964 the CMS monthly reports noted that the missionary at Numbulwar spoke on the dangers of smoking cigarettes and suggested that the shop order only pipe tobacco rather than cigarette tobacco (Church Missionary Society November 1964). In 1970 mission staff and Aboriginal Christians decided to collect and destroy cards to prevent gambling (Church Missionary Society January 1970).

With the advent of the Christian revival movements among Aborigines in the 1980s (which have had marked success in the region) and the complete Aboriginalisation of local churches, the local Christians preach and conduct their religious affairs independently and use Christianity as a vehicle of social control. At one Bible Camp I heard complaints that people were 'out fishing' and at their outstations instead of being present to enjoy 'fellowship' with their fellow Christians. The rigid stance by the early missions against the evils of drugs and gambling has been maintained over the years, and now Aboriginal Christians in the region also focus on petrol sniffing. Bos notes that the Yolngu Christian Revival movement of 1979 had been, in part, a Yolngu response to increasing problems of alcohol abuse and petrol sniffing (Bos 1988, 432). The Christian members of communities where petrol sniffing is practised say that they pray for the petrol sniffers. At Angurugu on Groote Eylandt a large number of sniffers (said to be more than fifty) took a pledge in the church grounds to give up their sniffing, an action which occurred in March 1988 on the eve of a visit by the Archbishop of Canterbury (*Northern Territory News* 4 March 1988). Some sniffers subsequently maintained their abstention and now refer to themselves as Christians; others have since relapsed. Aboriginal Christians in the region have composed a song which is said to have 'helped' the petrol sniffers. It goes:

I can't sniff petrol/drink beer/play cards;
This day
I'm going to see the King
Hallelulah! Hallelulah![2]

Influential church leaders preach directly on the subject of petrol sniffing. When the Archbishop of Canterbury visited, he was accompanied by the Aboriginal Bishop of Carpentaria from Yarrabah, Queensland (Bishop Arthur Malcolm), who gave a speech to the Aboriginal community:

> Here at this community I see young people walking around with soft drink cans in their hands, and we all know what's in those soft drink cans, and we must try to do something about it. Are we witnessing for Christ among our children? We have to make ourselves available for our children...take them out for the day, give them something to do. Teach them about our culture, how to hunt, how to fish. As I look around, nothing been happening. Sniffing petrol is a bad thing, it ruins people's lives.... . I've seen kids here who are skin and bone, because that thing is working in their body. We are part of the blame.... . Cry our hearts out now, and help them. Show them we love them.... . Every time we take a mouthful of beer one or two cells of our brain are killed. Same with petrol. The only way we can stop it is through Jesus Christ.... . I won't be tormented by the Devil, because I know where I stand with Christ. My advice to you, I ask you to really think about your young people...make sure the Church is doing something for them. These young ones have to carry on the Christian Gospel.[3]

Indeed, the Church claimed some success during this period. Apart from its regular Fellowship meetings, which attracted those already declaring themselves to be Christians, a youth movement involving dance routines to rock gospel songs took hold, and was said to have converted large numbers of young people including some who were petrol sniffers. The rock gospel movement is called 'Action'. The words of rhythmic rock gospel songs were choreographed into movement — primarily hand and arm movements — and performed in unison by mass assemblies of people arranged in rows. 'God aerobics' was how one amused white onlooker described it. The idea originated at Galiwin'ku on Elcho Island — also the location from which the earlier revival had sprung in 1979 (see Cole 1980, 98; Bos 1988). Early in 1988 at a thanksgiving weekend at Galiwin'ku, there had been 'a movement of the Spirit, a revival',[4] and 'Action' was conceived in its modern form (J Renata, personal communication):

Actions is an instrument of God. When they hear a song, they think of the meanings and put the Actions...in eighteen years I've never seen the youth movement so strong and to attract the adults. A Christian wants to help the total person — we are fighting a spiritual war. Action songs — they think it and it touches them, it touch their needs.

The Aboriginal minister declared at one Action session 'God really loved you when He gave you that Action'.

The driving rhythmic music (amplified over sophisticated electronic equipment) and the attraction of performing coordinated movement en masse took Aboriginal communities in the region by storm. On Groote Eylandt, by June 1988, Action had been performed every night without fail for two months — performances commenced at 6 pm (sometimes earlier) and continued until midnight involving up to 200 participants. The technique was transmitted by travelling demonstration teams and spread to Maningrida, Milingimbi, Yirrkala, Angurugu, Numbulwar and Ngukurr within months (see Brady 1989, 62). The teams chartered light aircraft in order to cover the region. New songs were choreographed over time using a simple technique of symbolic hand and arm movements to signify the words of the songs. 'Sin' is signed by crossed wrists (also Aboriginal sign

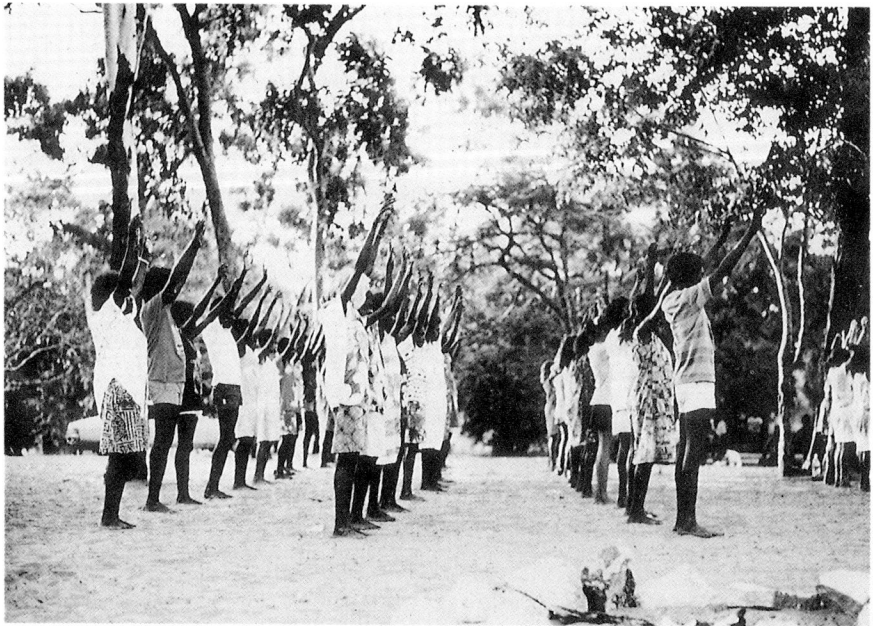

Plate 10: Young Christians perform Actions to rock gospel music in east Arnhem Land

language for gaol or police); 'Jesus' is upraised pointed arms; 'Jesus died' is arms outstretched as if on a cross; 'go' is signified by an outstretched arm describing a circle; 'love' is a hand on the heart. Women seated on the ground around the floodlit arena outside the church performed the movements where they sat; young toddlers were to be seen trying out the movements in their back gardens. Participants were primarily young people, men and women, aged from about five to thirty years. Action also attracted some young people who had previously sniffed petrol. An Aboriginal church leader in one of the communities influenced by Action in north-central Arnhem Land described how breakdancing had previously been popular but that the breakdancers had sniffed petrol. He said:

> We told them another dance with no problem — there's another way of bringing them out: Christian Action...some stopped sniffing, drinking kava and alcohol. Other sniffers followed them, came in and joined. R___ [his nephew] was leading that drama dance, drama actions.

He was also aware that 'conversion' did not always occur:

> Sniffers joined in, but not the hard core. They saw something new, the dancing. They [the sniffers] seems to be halfway now, they in the middle. At Fellowship, a sniffer hears and he tells

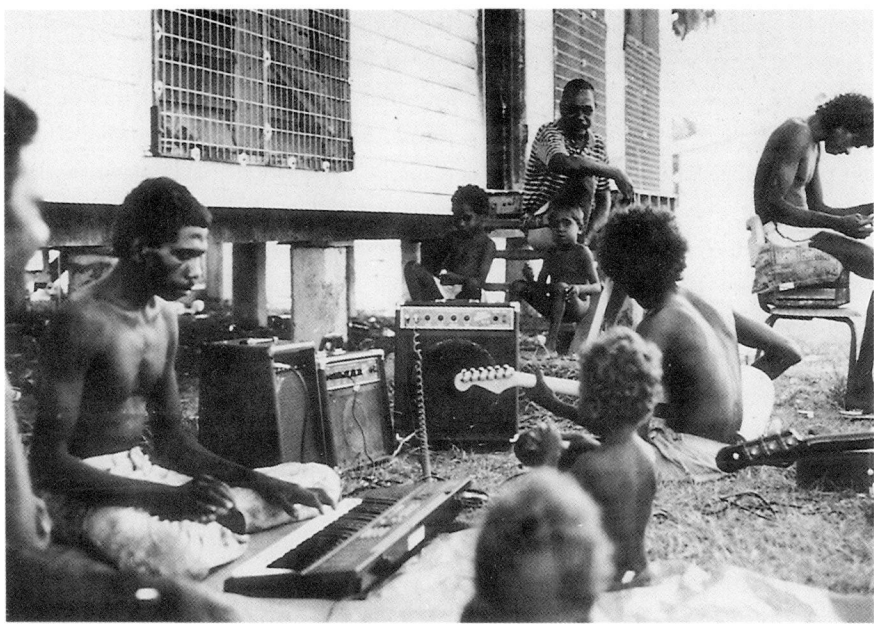

Plate 11: An informal Christian music session in north-central Arnhem Land, 1988

his friends he heard that story in Fellowship and start to interest. He look what is bad and what is good. They say they like to leave petrol; others pushing them. They find it difficult standing in between.

The personal account of one ex-sniffer stressed her sense of achievement through participation in Action:

> I always go to church, Fellowship. I'm number one for Action [ie the leader]...I was doing Action this year.... . When I was home back from hospital I didn't do any silly things [ie sniff] because I was doing well at Fellowship. They like me. I bin Christian. I bin baptised and confirmed in river. I'm good life, health, getting strong and too much tucker. I got good life and getting fat and strong. I bin forget about it, sniffing. I got a good Action.

It is clear that these mass movements, which achieve popularity to the degree of obsession, have tremendous power to influence, especially the young. People in the affected communities claimed that 'hundreds' of sniffers had given up the practice as a result. While such claims are probably exaggerated, Christian revivals aimed specifically at youth, and utilising music styles that appeal to that age group, come to offer an alternative network of friends and activities to those of the sniffing networks.[5] Those involved in Fellowship become surrounded by others who support their non-sniffing behaviour, and furthermore, they have a regular activity which consumes the hours which follow the closure of schools and work places. Some Aboriginal commentators frankly admitted that Action worked simply because it exhausted its participants: 'After Action the young ones get tired and go straight to bed. We ask them to stop getting cold [ie because they stay up late, they get cold] but they want more, so we carry on until they get knocked out!' Not everyone viewed this in a positive light. There were complaints from nursing sisters and school teachers that their staff left early in order to 'practise' their actions, and that younger children were tired in the mornings. Those who persisted in their petrol sniffing took delight in lurking around the performances in the dark, sometimes yelling out derisive comments and ironically mimicking the movements. On these occasions church people sometimes approached these young men and women and attempted dialogue with them. Direct engagement of this nature with sniffers was otherwise rare. The performances sometimes took on the appearance of a symbolic 'war', with the sniffers playing their own heavy metal cassettes loudly on the fringes of the Action arena, attempting to drown out the more modulated tones of Cliff Richard.

The Christians in general also provoked some criticism from non-participants, who claimed that while the adults attended their Bible Camps and evening Fellowships, their children were left unsupervised, sometimes to sniff petrol. One man said 'When they have service here and Bible Camp, all they're saying is 'love' and 'caring' but I don't know what they mean for that because they know what kids are doing and don't stop them'. At one community a Petrol Sniffing Committee was formed, with weekly meetings of approximately twelve Aborigines and four or five white staff. At one meeting, which coincided with a Fellowship meeting elsewhere in the settlement, several people wanted to go straightaway to the Christians and urge them to be more concerned about sniffing children and attend the committee meetings instead of prayer meetings. In turn, the Aboriginal minister tried to persuade the committee to meet during the day (which would have been less convenient) so it would not clash with his Fellowship gatherings.

Another facet of the interaction between Aboriginal Christians and petrol sniffing concerns attitudes towards physical punishment. Although physical punishment is on the whole disavowed by Aboriginal people, it does occur both in private and in public. Aboriginal Christians, however, express ethical and spiritual objections to spankings and beatings. This is ironic in view of the fact that when the CMS was in charge of these communities, the white missionaries engaged in physical punishment of Aboriginal children who misbehaved.[6] A Council chairman, apparently unaware of the contradiction, told me 'Christians are frightened about belting. The missionaries belted kids. Once J____ stole from the store and missionary belted him. Parents didn't argue [about this] with missionaries'. Christian women (brought up in the old Anglican mission) at one community said that they had solved the petrol-sniffing problem 'with love'. 'We prayed to the Lord and sniffing stopped; we gave them milk and talked to them.' Another woman provided her own interpretation of how to resolve the problem of being a Christian and the need for sniffers to be punished:

> They used a hose pipe to beat them on the bum, not [on the] back. You got to punish with love, don't show your anger, punish them proper way. If God sees us doing cruelty, He takes them away then. Have to deal with children with love. I called out [to the punishers] 'that's enough! You want to killem?'

PURITANICAL INFLUENCE IN THE WESTERN DESERT

The communities in Western Australia which were part of this study were established from 1934 onwards by the United Aborigines' Mission, an evangelical 'faith' mission of stern principles. These communities underwent a Christian revival in 1982, which, incidentally, was sparked as a result of contact with Galiwin'ku in the north (Stanton 1988, 303). The revival involved a 'Black Crusade' of ten

Aborigines who travelled from Warburton, Blackstone and the Musgrave Ranges to Mount Margaret, Leonora, Kalgoorlie and Wiluna among other locations (Morgan 1986, 290). The influence of this Aboriginal-led revival spread into South Australia (see Brady and Palmer 1988). At least one observer viewed the Crusade as having an impact on petrol sniffing: 'not that it did anything immediate for the kids but that it gave to their parents and the community a sense of hope, a sense that something good was happening in the community, and that had a profound effect for a time' (Marshall, Senate Select Committee 1985, 181). A Uniting Church worker observed that a Christian revival had somewhat tenuously dislodged sniffing in the Pitjantjatjara Lands in the early 1980s (Clark, Senate Select Committee 1985, 1457):

> The revival had seen them dramatically curtail the amount of open petrol sniffing. It seemed to be just under the surface and the people seemed to be taking a little more responsibility for the problem... . But, as one person said to me, it was like one of those little fires that is just burning under the brush, waiting for a big wind to come along to whip it away again.

Several Aboriginal men came to political prominence as a result of their leadership role in the Crusade, and still exert influence over community matters as a result. This has taken the form of a puritanical influence on several issues, some of which affect young people. For example, although most of the settlements in the region have had churches built — usually large airy structures with cement floors — only one settlement has a recreation hall which can be used for social functions by young people. The churches appear to be used rarely, but tentative suggestions from some quarters that they could be used for other purposes, such as film shows, have met with opposition from the Aboriginal Christian leaders. In one settlement an old church building was converted into a temporary store; but despite the construction of a new store, the building is to revert to a church, rather than becoming a recreation hall. The Christians have forbidden the use of the church buildings for any musical performances involving rock groups; indeed rock bands are few in the region, in marked contrast to Arnhem Land and eastern settlements. Christian musicians do play electric guitars and keyboards, but their use is restricted to a low-key accompaniment to the singing of Christian songs and hymns.

In short, adults who identify themselves as Christians frequently make decisions that prevent the development of youth activities which could help to deflect interest in petrol sniffing. The region is marked by poor recreational facilities for young people (in comparison with those available elsewhere), and so far the Christian groups have failed to offer petrol sniffers any viable movement with which they could identify. For individuals, their Christianity helps them to maintain sobriety and a non-smoking stance, and one young man who had been a chronic sniffer told me that he was now a Christian and played guitar for the regular Fellowship session. Others who described themselves as church people took a laissez-faire attitude. For example, one woman said that Christians lived together a good way, and did not fight, but she thought that Christianity could not help drinkers or petrol sniffers because 'that's their way'.

THE CRIMINALISATION OF PETROL SNIFFING

There have been several attempts at legal measures to make the sniffing of petrol, or the supply of petrol for the purpose of sniffing, an offence. To date, legislative measures of this order are in place in only two regions of Australia: in the Pitjantjatjara Lands in the northwest of South Australia and the Ngaanyatjarra Lands across the border in Western Australia. In all other areas where petrol sniffing is practised, the police may only take action if the individual is charged with an officially designated 'offence', such as break and enter, larceny or illegal use of a motor vehicle.

On occasions, state and territory governments come under pressure, both from Aboriginal people and from the police/judiciary, to make sniffing an offence. For example, in 1987 a test case on the supply of petrol to children for the purpose of sniffing was heard in a Darwin court under Section 154 of the Northern Territory Criminal Code. Three adult Aborigines (aged eighteen, twenty and twenty) were charged with supplying a potentially dangerous substance to children, and the prosecutor argued that 'this legislation must be used — there is nothing else available' (*Sunday Territorian* 25 January 1987). However, the magistrate found that there was no case to answer.

Until comparatively recently in Western Australia, petrol sniffers could be charged under Section 65 of the Western Australian Police Act which makes it an offence for 'every person having in his possession without lawful excuse, the proof of which shall be on such person, any deleterious drug'. Individuals found sniffing entered the justice system in this way, as well as through charges of disorderly conduct or as a result of other offences which they committed while intoxicated (Smith and McCulloch 1986, 1). The use of the 'deleterious drug' provision resulted in fourteen charges over a twelve-month period (recorded at Laverton) specifically for petrol sniffing. Juvenile offenders were all male, aged between twelve and seventeen. However, over the same period (July 1987– June 1988) offences associated with petrol sniffing (such as possession of a deleterious drug, threatening behaviour or breaking and entering) totalled forty-eight, committed by thirteen individual juveniles. Seventeen adults committed sixty offences associated with petrol sniffing in this period (Western Australian Police Department data, Laverton, 14 September 1988). Penalties for possession were fines (usually $50), community service orders, or placement in the care of the Department for Community Services.

The notable feature of these police figures is that a high number of offences were committed by only a few individuals. In one community two fifteen-year-old boys were charged with eleven offences. In another, only four charges were made over the twelve-month period, and all were against the same fifteen-year-old boy. The Department for Community Services in Western Australia expressed concern that 'a small group of chronic sniffers fell into a routine of arrest and removal to the Remand Centre followed by a return to the community only to be promptly re-arrested'. The department also disapproved of the 'use of the criminal system to solve a maladaptive health risk problem' (Smith and McCulloch 1986, 2). In 1988 the Western Australian Supreme Court ruled that unless a substance such as petrol or glue is distributed with a warning that it is deleterious (unless used for its prescribed purpose), the substance cannot be deemed deleterious. However, in July 1989, at the request of the Aboriginal communities in the area, by-laws were promulgated in the Ngaanyatjarra Lands of Western Australia creating offences in relation to the supply or use of deleterious substances for the purpose of inhalation.

In South Australia there are also by-laws under the Pitjantjatjara Land Rights Act 1981 which make it an offence to possess or supply petrol for the purpose of inhalation. These are discussed shortly. This area, now held under freehold title by Pitjantjatjara people who live in the northwest of South Australia (see Figure 11), has a history of legal remedies for petrol sniffing which place their recent legislative actions into perspective. In December 1970, the superintendent of what was then the North-West Reserve made a Superintendent's Order (which he was legally empowered to do) as follows (Hope 1983, 190):

> Petrol sniffing is prohibited at Amata and the whole of the North-West Reserve. Anyone found petrol sniffing may have to go to court and might have to pay a fine of $10. Children under the age of 18 will also have to go to court, but their parents may be asked to pay a large fine. If the fine were not paid a parent would have to go to gaol. By order of the Superintendent of the North-West Reserve.

The notion — promulgated by whites — that parents should be 'made' to take responsibility for the offences (petrol-sniffing related or otherwise) of their children had become apparent in 1969 when a magistrate dealt with a child offender by fining his mother. Fifteen years after this, the South Australian

Aboriginal Customary Law Committee (composed of a judge, a police officer and, significantly, an ex-superintendent of a North-West Reserve community) recommended (1984, 32):

> We consider that one of the most effective ways of so assisting adults would be to enjoin upon them legal responsibility for controlling their children. This may be, and has been, done through the courts, by requiring adults to be answerable for the delicts of their children.

The Committee went on to recommend that petrol sniffing be made an offence, and that in respect of children (seventeen years and under) convicted of the offence the penalties should be levied on either the child's mother, father, or person recognised by the Pitjantjatjara as standing in *loco parentis*. Penalties were recommended to be fines of between $100 and $500 (South Australian Customary Law Committee 1984, 84). No action was taken at a government level in response to these recommendations, but the Aboriginal population itself began to demand legal remedies. Having had the presence of petrol sniffing and associated offending behaviour and social disorder for twenty years (Worrall 1982), together with a series of largely unsuccessful and fragmented interventions, the Pitjantjatjara turned to the powers granted to them under state laws. In 1987 three by-laws were created by an Act to amend the Pitjantjatjara Land Rights Act, 1981, which ruled on the control of alcoholic liquor, the control of gambling and the control of petrol. The by-law governing petrol empowered police to confiscate and dispose of any petrol that they reasonably suspected was to be used or had been used for the purpose of inhalation and any container that contained or had contained petrol (Pitjantjatjara Land Rights (Control of Petrol) By-Laws 1987). A person could be charged with possessing, selling or supplying petrol for the purpose of inhalation, the maximum penalty for supplying being a $2,000 fine or imprisonment for up to two years.

One of the reasons for implementing these by-laws was that previously the police had no powers to take away petrol sniffers' cans (this would constitute 'assault'); in addition, the by-laws enable the magistrates (who hear cases on their circuit court visits to the Pitjantjatjara Lands) to make a variety of orders regarding the treatment or rehabilitation of sniffers. In reality, there are few options apart from fines and good behaviour bonds. There has been only one 'rehabilitation program' available since 1987, the counselling work undertaken by the Healthy Aboriginal Life Team (HALT). In a sample of forty-one petrol-sniffing offences in the Pitjantjatjara Lands (over approximately twelve months) thirty-four males and seven females were charged with possession, supply or sale of petrol under the by-laws. The majority (twenty-five) were fined amounts ranging from $50 to $200, while six were referred to the HALT team. In the remaining cases, the charges were dismissed without penalty, warrants were issued for non-appearance at court and good behaviour bonds ordered (Pitjantjatjara Council files).[7] The by-laws do not allow for action to be taken if a sniffer is found intoxicated in possession of an empty container, and the Pitjantjatjara are lobbying for the inclusion of petrol within the Public Intoxication Act (South Australia).[8] This would mean that the police could apprehend an intoxicated sniffer, process him or her at the police station or take the individual home to parents. Many Anangu (Pitjantjatjara Aborigines) believe that these would be useful additional provisions, as at present

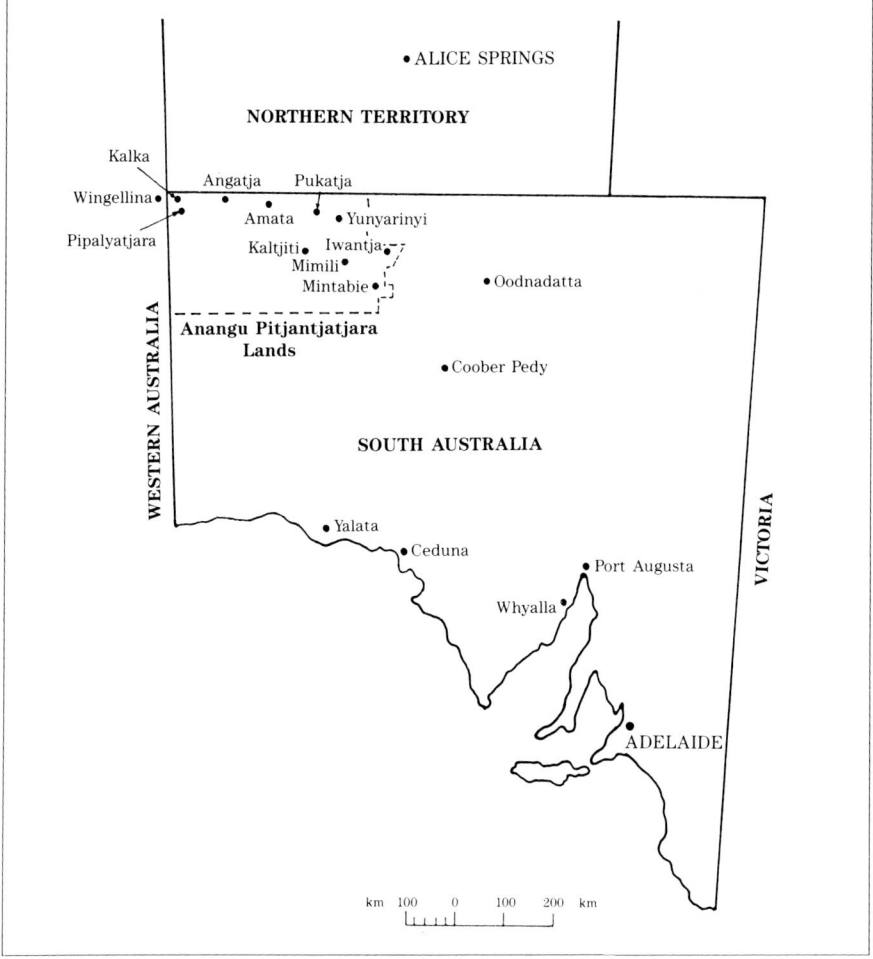

Figure 11: Anangu Pitjantjatjara Lands on the border of South Australia, Western Australia and the Northern Territory

the police are unwilling to apprehend sniffers (a situation complicated by police concerns as a result of the Royal Commission into Aboriginal Deaths in Custody).[9]

Any reliance on these measures, however, signifies that there is an unwillingness on the part of Aboriginal people to commit themselves to direct intervention. In effect, they have conceded that they are unable to act effectively and have stated strongly that 'white' law has to be implemented. Some communities in the region have expressed the wish that petrol sniffers appear at court, and some have also reiterated the view that the parents of sniffers be taken to court (M Tehan, personal communication). As we have seen, this idea was instigated by a white magistrate twenty years ago. At their Council meetings, the Pitjantjatjara express the view that they wish to enforce, and concentrate on, Anangu Law (ie traditional religious law), and thus by implication suggest that sniffing does not fall under its rubric, but under white law. White law has a strong presence on the lands — there are seventeen police officers and Aboriginal 'police aides' on or near the lands, with a police headquarters at Marla Bore in the east. Four communities have two Aboriginal aides each, with their own police vehicles and uniforms. Aboriginal residents have themselves requested this enlarged police presence, and complained in previous years that the police were too far away (at Oodnadatta) and thus unable to respond rapidly to calls (South Australian Aboriginal Customary Law Committee 1984, 125). In this instance, their expressed wishes were acted upon.

Whether or not the policing of their lands and the implementation of legal remedies for petrol sniffing has had the desired effect of 'restoring into the hands of parents authority to control their children' (South Australian Aboriginal Customary Law Committee 1984, 90) is another matter. It could be argued that these actions serve to reinforce the notion that petrol sniffing is the responsibility of whites rather than Aborigines (even if eight Aboriginal police aides participate in the enactment of the laws). On the other hand, if 'citizens' of Australia, be they Aboriginal or white, have a 'real problem' and are 'calling for assistance' as the committee indicated, then presumably the government has a responsibility to respond accordingly. In keeping with this view, one welfare officer in the Northern Territory (Sargent 1977, 6) stated unequivocally:

> I do not agree with the very common attitude that because these are problems of the Aboriginal people that they (the Aboriginals) have to find the answers. I see this as an excuse by the authorities responsible to abdicate that responsibility and involvement; and they do it under the very admirable guise of 'self-determination'.

Nevertheless, the situation described above raises some difficult questions relating to Aboriginal self-management — after all, the official government response to petrol sniffing states that 'actions in response to petrol sniffing should originate from and be controlled by the Aboriginal people' (Commonwealth of Australia 1985, 220). It may be that the increased police and judicial involvement in petrol sniffing was indeed an Aboriginal-instigated move, even though it represents the wishes of people who have, through institutionalisation over the years, adopted non-Aboriginal solutions which were demonstrated to them by the superintendent of their reserve. But what of other suggestions emanating from 'Aboriginal communities'? Some suggest that sniffers' parents be imprisoned for not looking after their children properly, and that the sniffers should all be 'sent away'. These too are the wishes of Aboriginal people themselves which should logically be acknowledged and acted upon. There are indeed some dangers in desperation, for communities may grasp at magical solutions involving the police, incarceration, foster homes and institutions, and scare tactics because such interventions absolve them of taking responsibility for their own youth (Brady 1985a, 7).

As petrol sniffing is not an offence in jurisdictions other than the South Australian Pitjantjatjara Lands and the Western Australian Ngaanyatjarra Lands, it is difficult to assess the extent to which petrol sniffers commit other offences and come to the attention of the judicial system. Certainly many observers have noted a high association between offending behaviour (officially designated as such) and sniffing (Worrall 1982; Tomlinson 1975; Sargent 1977; Eastwell 1979), although a study in South Australia found that offenders tended to be older than petrol sniffers within the juvenile age range (Brady and Morice 1982). Some have commented that it is only when sniffers engage in other 'criminal' activities that any notice is taken of them by Aborigines and non-Aborigines alike (Tomlinson 1975; Hayward-Ryan 1979; Elsegood nd).

Other than giving the petrol sniffer a period of abstinence from petrol, regular meals and providing the home community with a break from persistently offending sniffers, incarceration does not seem to have any rehabilitative impact on sniffers. Their health and physical fitness undoubtedly improves, and community members frequently observe that sniffers who offend return from gaol looking fat and healthy. The provision of weightlifting equipment in one gaol has probably been responsible for an acceleration of interest in body building among Aboriginal young men in the Northern Territory, and some of their home communities have followed up this interest and purchased weights in an attempt to provide diversionary recreational facilities.

An alternative to traditional incarceration in the Northern Territory is an initiative which deserves mention. In 1986 the Northern Territory Department of Correctional Services established a 'wilderness work camp' for repeated juvenile offenders, along the lines of an Outward Bound program. This has become known as Wildman River, named after its location 160 kilometres east of Darwin. The detainees engage in a strenuous program of physical fitness and work, learning basic skills such as welding and carpentry. As a Northern Territory government publication announced, 'At Wildman River bad boys learn to become good men, the hard way' (Northern Territory Digest 1988). The Wildman River scheme inevitably receives some offenders whose misdeeds are associated with petrol sniffing. In the Northern Territory, these constituted 9.4 per cent of all juvenile offences between January 1986 and June 1989 (see Table 9 below).

Table 9: Juvenile offences associated with substance abuse, January 1986 – June 1989

	Number
Petrol-sniffing related offences	131 (9.4% of total)
Drugs	23
Alcohol	175
Glue sniffing	7
Unknown	153
Not related to substance abuse	905
Total clients	1,393

(Source: Northern Territory Correctional Services)

Table 10: Petrol-sniffing related offences by age and sex, Northern Territory, January 1986 – June 1989

Age	13	14	15	16	17	Total
Male	2	12	11	51	33	109 (83.2%)
Female	1		1	13	7	22 (16.8%)
Total	3	12	12	64	40	131

(Source: Northern Territory Correctional Services)

The detainees at Wildman River are all male, and are generally aged between fifteen and seventeen. As Table 10 shows, petrol-sniffing related offences in the Northern Territory are predominantly committed by males, with ninety-five such offences in the fifteen to seventeen age bracket. All were Aboriginal and the most common offence related to sniffing was break and enter. Not all these offenders would be detained at Wildman River (it holds eighteen people

Table 11: Petrol-sniffing related offences, from most to least serious, and by age and sex, January 1986 – June 1989 (female figures in brackets)

Type of offence	\	Age of juvenile				
	13	14	15	16	17	Total
Assault			1	2	2	5
			(0)	(0)	(0)	(0)
Sex offences					1	1
					(0)	(0)
Break and enter	2	7	11	37	23	80
	(0)	(0)	(1)	(9)	(4)	(14)
Stealing	1	2		8	4	15
	(1)	(0)		(0)	(0)	(1)
Justice procedures				3	2	5
				(0)	(1)	(1)
Motor vehicle related		2		7	5	14
		(0)		(0)	(2)	(2)
Property damage				3	1	4
				(1)	(0)	(1)
Receiving				2	1	3
				(2)	(0)	(2)
Weapon-related					1	1
					(0)	(0)
Trespass			1	2		3
			(0)	(1)		(1)
Total	3	12	12	64	40	131
	(1)	(0)	(1)	(13)	(7)	(22)

(Source: Northern Territory Correctional Services)

comfortably), and some transfer between other established detention centres. By May 1988 the camp had had seventy-three admissions, 79 per cent of whom were Aboriginal, drawn primarily from the northern regions of the Northern Territory, although 12 per cent were from Central Australia. The rate of recorded re-offenders was 33 per cent, which is somewhat lower than the average for the territory (Mason and Wilson 1988, 103–7). The camp is a rugged experience and has a strong emphasis on physical fitness and hard work — there is a daily fifteen-kilometre run. It takes up to two months before the boys are fit enough to perform the rest of the work routine (Mason and Wilson 1988, 104). In order to be classified as suitable for the camp, a doctor assesses each juvenile (Northern Territory Correctional Services, personal communication). In addition all juveniles admitted to any detention centre have blood tests taken, including blood lead levels. The scheme has the advantage of being more economical to the Northern Territory government (approximately $70–$80 a day compared with $100 a day in a conventional institution). It is also a desirable alternative to prison. Aboriginal youths of fifteen and sixteen are frequently incarcerated in the 'adult' gaol in Darwin, where there are no special programs available for them (Northern Territory Correctional Services, personal communication).

POLICING

As mentioned earlier, police officers in some regions express frustration that they have few powers to apprehend petrol sniffers unless an offence is committed. As the years pass, and sniffing appears to remain entrenched in certain communities, Aboriginal people too, often express the opinion that the police should be 'doing something'. On occasions Aboriginal people ask the police to 'flog' sniffers, but such corporal punishment is beyond their official powers. Others feel that the police could help in more informal ways; for example, an Aboriginal member of the State Working Party on Petrol Sniffing in Western Australia believed the police had a role in his home community. He thought they should round up the sniffers and bring them to community meetings, so that 'the community could talk to them, say encouraging words — not 'You rubbish kids' in front of parents, but 'We brought you here to tell you petrol sniffing is dangerous and some of the families done the wrong thing by speaking up for you. In this way, we're trying to help you".

This reference to the families 'speaking up' for sniffers relates to problems in the region in which parents step in to defend their sons or daughters against community attempts to chastise or intervene in their actions. In these instances it is clear that community members place some weight on the role of official representatives of the law, who are non-Aboriginal, and outsiders. Their separation from the interlocking relationships of the communities allows them to act without grumbling and retribution from the relatives of offenders. It is ironic that while concerned white liberals and Aboriginal activists call for the police to temper the level of their interactions with Aborigines, some communities in remote areas are complaining that the police do not intervene more often, and urge that their powers be extended rather than curtailed.

Many police officers stationed in Aboriginal communities (as they are in parts of the Northern Territory) believe strongly that the incarceration of 'ringleaders' has a beneficial effect on the level of sniffing. Many written and anecdotal accounts assert that older, experienced petrol sniffers introduce and maintain the practice among others. Elsegood observed that young children are coopted by older sniffers as a means of obtaining petrol from areas otherwise inaccessible because of body size (Elsegood nd, 3). An Arnhem Land Council chairman to whom I spoke could name the five young men he said were the leaders: 'They lead the others, they share it out…if we could get them out [of the community] it would be better. They're not interested in sport, nothing. They want to pull this sport and recreation down.' The five young men he named were aged between sixteen and twenty-three. Of the twenty-one regular users of petrol in the community, twelve were aged between twenty and twenty-six; nine aged between fifteen and nineteen. So in this community, the 'leaders' were not notably older than their 'followers'. Although it is clear that the presence of particular individuals does seem to influence the level of sniffing, at least in some communities, it is not at all clear why this should be so. The notion of 'leaders' may be a convenient fiction upon which undue emphasis is placed — frequently by Europeans and the police — for example, Folds's notion of the 'king sniffer' (1987, 70).[10] It is similar in conception to the idea popular in non-Aboriginal society that there are drug 'pushers' — a theory which has been somewhat deflated by recent work suggesting that new recruits to heroin use (for example) often try the substance as a result of normal social associations with other users (often friends), rather than confrontations with unscrupulous dealers (Pearson 1987). Another factor which militates against the leader theory of petrol sniffing is the deep-seated objection to being 'bossed' on the part of many Aboriginal groups. The matter of age or status-graded differential associations among young men is also significant. In desert regions, it is unusual for young men past the occasion of their ritual entry into manhood to associate with immature 'boys'. It is also unlikely that one or two individuals would influence 'the sniffers' unless these people already formed part of his or her using group. The using groups are fluid and their membership changes over time, in keeping with other 'action' or 'task' groups which are convened informally for various activities (see Sansom 1980).

One final point which is neglected in the discussions about the ostensible influence of ringleaders is that many ex-sniffers I spoke to emphasised their personal choice to experiment with, and then to abandon, sniffing. 'I wanted to try it', they say. Their parents would naturally prefer to believe that 'other' boys persuaded them.

It is more likely that influential associates provoke sniffing by example, rather than through overt persuasion, in contradiction of the conventional view that ringleaders push the uninitiated into experimentation. For example, while attempting to understand the causes of the abandonment of the practice over a six-month period in one community, I discovered that a boy nominated by several observers, including the police, as being the 'main one', and thought to be absent from the community during the diminution of sniffing, was in fact present during this time. He was present but he had ceased to sniff petrol, as had all other users still present. He and others merely said they had 'decided' to stop. In this case, the cessation was due, in part, to the fact that a well-known user decided not to engage in sniffing, and by example had an influence on other regular users. When he recommenced, they did so too. Zinberg (1984) states that the setting, composed, in part, of the nature of the using group (whether it is controlled or compulsive), is influential. As Pearson (1987, 84) notes, friends are influential in either direction:

> It would be wrong to think of these contexts of friendship as only concerning 'bad company' which can lead people astray. Friendship can be both the route into certain kinds of drug choices, and also the way out. And even within a single friendship network, different people will nevertheless exercise different options and at different times.

'THE WELFARE'

Government welfare officers sometimes involve themselves in the petrol-sniffing issue, either through their advocacy role when juveniles attend court hearings, or through direct consultation with the families of children using petrol. They have the power to compile social background reports which should ideally document the familial circumstances perceived as being antecedent to the court appearance (Brady 1985b), and to recommend penalties to the courts. These may involve incarceration, fostering, or placement in a variety of homes or rehabilitation centres. As a result of the history of the role of the welfare bureaucracy in the forcible division of Aboriginal families, and particularly the removal of mixed-descent children from their parents, welfare officers are still viewed with apprehension by many Aboriginal people. This suspicion makes their contemporary role a delicate and difficult one. An illuminating example of present sensitivities towards official government intervention occurred during my research in an Arnhem Land settlement. A local welfare officer, herself of Aboriginal descent, attempted to compile some useful data on the petrol sniffers and their families. She started to administer a questionnaire which asked caregivers how they felt about the child's behaviour, whether the child had been to court, and what interventions, if any, the adults had attempted. She was forced to abandon the questionnaire because she received such a hostile reception. A subsequent head office memorandum observed (Northern Territory Department of Health and Community Services report 1988):

> Most caregivers initially stated that their children did not sniff petrol...others stated that they had done something about it. [The welfare officer] believed that all caregivers felt ashamed and very embarrassed that they were being questioned. Many were reluctant to answer questions. The most common and biggest fear of caregivers appeared to be that welfare were going to remove their children.

This revealing incident demonstrates much about Aboriginal responses to direct confrontation (even of a low-key nature and by a known individual) about petrol sniffing. Nevertheless, the intervention — albeit a curtailed and misinterpreted one — by a representative of the welfare bureaucracy was probably responsible, along with a series of other factors (including the increased use of kava, the popularity of Christian Action and the dry season), for a diminution of petrol sniffing in that community which persisted for six months.

LOCAL INITIATIVES

Between 1979 and 1981 researchers from the School of Medicine at the Flinders University of South Australia (including myself) undertook studies at a community on the far west coast of the state. Yalata is associated with the Pitjantjatjara and Yankuntjatjara communities in the far northwest of South Australia, with Ngaanyatjarra-speaking people and with Cundeelee (now Coonana) in Western Australia. Yalata experienced a rise in petrol sniffing in 1976, although sporadic use had occurred before this. The research team collected blood samples from as many young people as possible within the ten to seventeen age group: sixty-two individuals aged between ten and seventeen in 1979 (forty-one boys and twenty-one girls). Of these, twenty individuals had, in 1979, used enough petrol to elevate their blood lead levels above 20 micrograms per decilitre (seventeen boys and three girls). Their mean age was 14.55 years. Others used petrol occasionally so that nineteen showed lead levels of between 10 and 20 micrograms per decilitre.

Throughout the late 1970s and early 1980s there were virtually no local sanctions in place aimed at the petrol sniffers in this community. Those who offended, and whose offences were reported, were processed by the juvenile justice system (see Brady 1985b). Some were incarcerated in an institution in Adelaide. Occasionally, at the instigation of the school, a community advisor or the magistrate, the residents were coerced into a public admonishment of some description. On one occasion the sniffers were given a public hiding by unwilling parents and other relatives. On another, they were lined up before the magistrate and an assembled audience in the local hall. Some wept with shame. At the time no deaths had occurred and no sniffers showed marked physical symptoms, although some had fits and showed jerky and uncoordinated movements. By 1988, five people from the original cohort of sixty-two had died: three males (two from petrol-sniffing causes and one from unknown causes); and two females (one as the result of violence, the other from heart disease). Of the original cohort, deducting the five deceased individuals, eight were sniffing petrol in 1988, nine years later. These were six males and two females, having a mean age of twenty-two years.

At Yalata in 1988 there were also ten other users of petrol, who participated in a locally initiated 'sniffer's camp', located some kilometres from the settlement, supervised by an Aboriginal married couple. These were mostly younger people. The camp infrastructure was funded by the South Australian Drug and Alcohol Services Council, and the supervisors were paid from Community Development Employment Program (CDEP) funds. The provision of the camp (and the relative isolation of its clients) went hand-in-hand with the provision of attractive activities in the settlement — therefore there was some positive reinforcement for users to give up the practice or else be excluded out at the sniffers' camp. The sniffers' camp residents were also taken up to an outstation northwest of Maralinga on at least one occasion. By way of contrast to the somewhat romantic notion that a sojourn at an outstation is somehow inherently 'rehabilitative', it was salutary to observe the activities of the young clients in February 1988 at a location in the Great Victoria Desert. The adolescent boys appeared to be at a loose end: they cut down branches and made themselves a large shade with tarpaulins; one had a cassette player and so they sat under their shade listening to music. Some obtained the keys of the outstation tractor and drove it around. One of their supervisors arranged for them to clean up rubbish around the camps one morning, and two came with a colleague and myself and others on a hunting trip. They were inexperienced in the techniques of dealing appropriately with hunted red kangaroo. The group appeared to eat virtually no bush food during their stay, having come handsomely provisioned with boxes of canned products, on which they all gorged. Several attempted to hitch rides back to the settlement (five hours away), and altogether appeared relieved to be leaving when the time came. Few adults already at the outstation made any effort to interact with the adolescents or involve them in the day's activities.

Despite the development of sniffing among some younger people, the practice dwindled towards the end of 1988 and for the first time in some twelve years, the community has been relatively free of petrol sniffing. The clinic reported no emergency management of sniffing-related symptoms over a two-year period (1987–89). A Yalata youth who had been away from the community for twelve months died in Adelaide in July 1988 from petrol-related causes (see Chapter Four, Table 5). The decline of sniffing has probably been partly due to the provision of a flexible system of funding which enables a range of local Aborigines to be paid as 'youth workers' who take responsibility for providing activities for adolescents. The youth program focussed on general activities, including sports, hunting, discos and camps. The community employed one worker funded by what was then the Department of Aboriginal Affairs and four workers under the CDEP scheme. All the positions except for the coordinator's were flexible and were filled by Yalata residents. Other funding agencies involved included the state Department for Community Welfare (which provided $2,500 for equipment) and the Drug and Alcohol Services Council (which funded the substance abuse component). Because of savings made at Yalata, this funding was spread over an extra two years. The next project is to obtain funds for a building to house sports activities. For a community which suffers from heavy alcohol use at times, has a long history of ill-conceived government intervention, and a population which consciously avoided direct sanctions against sniffing, the present diminution in petrol sniffing at Yalata is a notable success.[11]

SOCIAL RESTRAINTS

Petrol-using groups in some regions are now aware of institutionalised objections to the practice of petrol sniffing. These are most marked in the Pitjantjatjara and Ngaanyatjarra Lands, where the communities themselves have insisted on making sniffing, and the supply of petrol for the purpose of sniffing, an offence under their by-laws. Whatever the historical and social context from which this sanction has arisen, the decision makes it clear that the community residents want action to prevent sniffing, and the sniffers in those communities are now on the defensive since their activities can provoke an appearance at court or involvement with the police. Sniffers and their families are also uncomfortably aware that welfare workers are alarmed about the practice, and because of the historical associations between 'the welfare' and the removal of children from their homes, this has, in some cases, provoked a response.

There has been considerable animated discussion about the role of policing and incarceration as incitement or deterrent to the practices of sniffing and offending which will not be reiterated here (Biles 1983; Gilroy 1976). Whether or not detention is a pleasant or an unpleasant experience is hard to say without some in-depth investigation, and responses probably depend upon a wide variety of circumstances. In view of the social advantages conferred on sniffers by identification with the mores of the sniffing culture, it is unlikely that incarceration in itself is the reforming agent it purports to be. The Wildman River work camp is more likely to produce beneficial outcomes if new associations are formed by its clientele which extend beyond sniffing preoccupations, and if detainees acquire new outlets (in the form of skills) which could introduce them to different social and work networks on their return to the home community. Pride in having a strong, muscled body may also act as a deterrent to the recommencement of sniffing.

From the user's point of view, increasing the level of anxiety associated with use (if, indeed, anxiety is evoked by these formal institutionalised sanctions) may serve to enhance the aura of danger already associated with petrol sniffing, and may affect the quality of the intoxication experience, making it more uncomfortable and negative. Nevertheless, as Zinberg (1984) and Watson (1987) suggest, external social controls are important. Zinberg (1984, 111–12) comments:

> The decision to use [an illicit psychedelic drug] brings great[er] anxiety because of the drug's greater promise of pleasure or pain.... Yet the social factor — the setting variable — should not be disregarded. The importance of setting showed up most strikingly among our controlled opiate users who, with the exception of those few who had an unusually well-developed system of internal checks, could not have remained controlled on the basis of personality factors alone. Instead, their ability to continue moderate use depended to a significant degree on social sanctions and rituals.... At the same time, however, they felt the anxiety engendered by society's association of opiate use with degradation, deviance and criminality.

In the contemporary Aboriginal context there is still a serious disjunction between formal and informal sanctions, which inhibits the development of a coherent and sensitive approach to the establishment of a setting that could serve to discourage use of petrol as an inhalant. Concerned individual Aborigines, some of whom had devoted themselves to the 'war on the sniffers' to the point of nervous and physical exhaustion, were disheartened by the pervasive lack of support and cooperation from the rest of the population. While the police and their appointed agents can act without retribution, and indeed are constantly urged in this direction by Aboriginal people, local efforts at prevention and control often meet with resistance, anger and outrage which undermine their success. While young people who engage in petrol sniffing know that their kin will publicly support them, taking their part against other community members, the fact that they may meet an officer of the police is of subsidiary concern. If, however, a consensus of community opinion becomes effectively mobilised to disapprove of sniffers' activities, to make them so uncomfortable and isolated that users desire reintegration into the larger society, then a combination of social and legal sanction may provide the framework for large-scale abandonment of the practice.

NOTES

1. Thanks to Dr V Burbank for this verbatim account (8 June 1988) from her fieldnotes.

2. Thanks to Dr V Burbank (personal communication) for this detail.

3. From a taped speech by Bishop Arthur Malcolm, Angurugu, 28 February 1988, recorded by Dr J Waddy, linguist, Angurugu.

4. Personal communication from J Renata, Nungalinya College, Darwin. The 1979 revival on Elcho Island was marked by nightly Fellowship, as well as communal singing. Bos (1988, 428) notes that 'many were action songs' and observed the acting out or 'dancing' with arm and body movements which took place, suggesting similarities with traditional ceremonial forms of dance.

5. Electric guitars and amplifiers are used by Christian music groups, but in one of those communities drum kits were said to be 'not allowed' in live music sessions. In another location drums were used.

6. Physical punishment, as well as other punitive techniques (shaving heads, forcing wrong-doers to wear flour sacks, the washing out of mouths with soapy water) were common practices among many denominations, not just the CMS, in the 1930s and 1940s.

7. I am grateful to legal advisers, Maureen Tehan and Richard Bradshaw, for their assistance with these data. In the region there have also been several attempts to establish working camps for sniffers and a youth counsellor was based in one settlement. These data are held in the Pitjantjatjara Council offices in Alice Springs.

8. This refers to individuals under the influence of a drug or alcohol. Petrol would need to be declared a 'drug' under the Act.

9. This is because 'processing' may involve a period of incarceration, and police have been advised by their state commissioner that those 'at risk' should not be locked up. The risk, in this instance, refers to that of suicide in custody (Commonwealth of Australia 1991).

10. One problem with Folds's analysis is that he rarely provides sources for his data; readers are unclear whether he has personally observed activities or heard second-hand descriptions.

11. The assistance of Richard Aspinall and Chloe Muller, who provided me with details of recent develoments, is gratefully acknowledged. I also made follow-up visits to Yalata and its outstation in 1990 and 1991.

CHAPTER

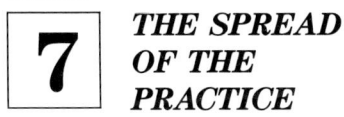

7 THE SPREAD OF THE PRACTICE

THE HISTORY OF PETROL SNIFFING

NORTHERN AUSTRALIA

The practice of sniffing petrol in order to alter mood has been known among Aboriginal people in northern Australia for approximately forty years. Its history elsewhere is longer; the earliest known report of the deliberate inhalation of petrol fumes is from the United States, in 1934 (Nunn and Martin 1934). In Australia, it is commonly believed that petrol sniffing among Aborigines started during the Second World War when large numbers of American servicemen were stationed throughout north Australia, in Queensland and the Northern Territory (Nurcombe et al 1970, 369; Senate Select Committee 1985, 1494).[1] Some would have it that the practice was initiated by Black Americans.

Often isolated in difficult physical conditions, so the story goes, some of these men inhaled petrol when other substances such as alcohol were unavailable. Aborigines are thought (presumably) to have taken up the practice in imitation. This piece of conventional wisdom is hard to verify and it is tempting to interpret it as an example of externalising blame — or of racism. Certainly there were large numbers of American (and Canadian) servicemen in north Australia during the war. In 1942, for example, 3,500 Black American troops were stationed at Mt Isa and 5,000 men were in the Darwin–Adelaide River region (Powell 1988; Hall 1980). No Black American troops were stationed anywhere along the coasts; all were in transport units further south (A Powell, personal communication). It is also true that the servicemen had an exceptional fondness for alcohol; this is documented by Powell who states that the men 'drank whatever they could get at whatever price' (1988, 204). Liquor was also stolen and home brews such as 'Mountain Dew' were concocted (Burd et al 1987). Powell (1988, 205) quotes Dennis Monger:

> It 'wasn't bad', he says, if you drilled a hole in a coconut, emptied a little milk out, put in raisins, rice and two spoonsful of torpedo alcohol, then bunged up the hole in the coconut and put it under the bed for three months. If it hadn't gone 'bang' by then 'you could have a rip-roaring night — and a hell of a headache the next morning'. Brews, it seems, were confined only by the availability of alcohol and the limits of human imagination.

Drinking, gambling, brawling and general 'lawlessness' were common among Australian and American troops (Mt Isa and Tennant Creek received particular mention in this context), as was sexual contact between servicemen and Aboriginal women (Powell 1988). But nowhere in these accounts is there any mention of the use of petrol as an inhalant. Indeed, historian Alan Powell, who had access to wartime medical reports and other documents, as well as having interviewed numerous American ex-servicemen, had never heard reference to petrol sniffing among these men (A Powell, personal communication).[2] The theory that sniffing was introduced by servicemen is certainly feasible, for fuel dumps and aircraft bases were scattered across northern coasts from Townsville to Port Hedland, and included several bases at Aboriginal missions: Groote Eylandt, Gove, Milingimbi and Port Keats, among others. While many mixed-descent Aborigines were evacuated south during the war, able-bodied men and 'full-bloods' remained (Powell 1988, 262), many involved in coastwatch networks and other roles associated with the armed forces. Nevertheless, several inquiries made of ex-servicemen and missionaries of the era have produced no confirmation. A serviceman stationed at the Umbakumba flying-boat base (Groote Eylandt) between 1939 and 1941 wrote (RN Torrington, personal communication):

> I was a friend of Fred Gray (who started Umbakumba) and often spent my days off at his home where there was a floating Aboriginal population of some fifty or more. I am sure that this subject would have come up, but I can say with assurance that this matter was unknown at that time...the Shell Company had approximately 1000 44 gallon drums of aviation fuel in a fuel dump backing onto the bush and it would have been extremely easy to tamper with these drums but I never heard of any comments in this regard.

The Reverend Keith Cole, historian for the CMS, wrote (personal communication):

> That it was started by servicemen — American or Australian — would seem to have no basis at all in fact. It seems to have started about the same time that people became aware of wide drug abuse among young non-Aboriginal people in the rest of Australia... . Certainly I have no record of petrol sniffing by Aboriginal people in any Top End community until well after World War II.

The earliest documented instance of Aboriginal people sniffing petrol in the Top End can be found in a report dated July 1950 by Patrol Officer Gordon Sweeney (Australian Archives: CA 1078 Native Affairs Branch, CRS: F315; 1949/393 A111).[3] Sweeney undertook a patrol and census at Lee Brothers sawmill, on the Cobourg Peninsula northeast of Darwin, where he found 108 Aborigines at the mill (fifty men, thirty-one women and twenty-seven children). About twenty of the men were employed at the mill. Sweeney inquired into several matters including 'Item 6. Natives inhaling petrol fumes'. His report notes briefly, 'The petrol at the mill is now locked up out of the way of natives disposed to inhale the fumes'. His census is significant, for it provides the names and 'tribes' of the Aborigines present, showing that they were of a variety of language groups drawn from a wide area of the north.

Some of the Aboriginal people Sweeney named in 1950 have been identified as now living at Oenpelli, Maningrida, Milingimbi, Croker Island, Melville Island and Goulburn Island.[4] The sawmill, established in the 1920s, acted as a 'focus of population drawing people from as far afield as Cape Don and the Liverpool River' (Peterson and Tonkinson 1979). When people dispersed throughout Arnhem Land in subsequent years, they took with them the knowledge of what they had seen. A Milingimbi man, whom I spoke to at Maningrida in 1989, had worked at Lee Brothers sawmill in 1956. He remembered that there had been petrol sniffing at Milingimbi in approximately 1950, and volunteered the view that it had been 'learnt' at the sawmill. Some of the communities to which these individuals returned still have a high prevalence of petrol sniffing, though Milingimbi is now free of it. A younger man, living at Maningrida, believed (personal communication):

> It started from Goulburn, they taught us. I was eight or nine [ie approximately 1968]. The sawmill in early days. People told me about the Lee Brothers sawmill and sniffing. People moved backwards and forwards to bush, had ceremonies there. Milingimbi, Goulburn, Ramingining, Maningrida, Oenpelli, all of a sudden spreading [ie sniffing] from Goulburn Island back to here.[5]

Petrol was not readily available in the 1950s, indeed the missions in the Arnhem Land region were usually short of vehicles. After the war, the army auctioned their trucks very cheaply and these 'blitz trucks' were often the first four-wheel drive vehicles available to anyone. Buffalo shooters and other small operators purchased them. Oenpelli, for example, only possessed one vehicle and a tractor before the war (R Levitus, personal communication). Sawmilling operations, however, needed petrol for their machinery (Mack 1985) and in 1956 for example, over seventy Aborigines were employed in the Darwin and Katherine regions in the timber industry, excluding mission-based enterprises (Sweeney 1956). Keith Hart, a CMS missionary at Oenpelli, reported that in approximately 1950 they had to drain the petrol out of the mission's sawbench because petrol sniffers were stealing it (K Hart, personal communication).

Judging by these early accounts, there was a hiatus between the first reports dated around 1950, and the beginnings of a more concentrated (and publicly notable) interest in the practice (see Figure 12). Nurcombe and others who published the first Australian academic account of the practice in 1970 noted that petrol sniffing had been in existence for ten years (since 1960) at Galiwin'ku on Elcho Island (Nurcombe et al 1970). An individual identified to me by health workers to be the 'first leader' of petrol sniffing at Maningrida was only born in 1959 and presumably did not experiment until he was at least eight or ten years old, dating its commencement there at 1967 or 1968. This individual was said to have 'learned in Darwin, and he brought it in. There was a second follower from a Ramingining man...they teach him how to sniff...he was the leader of the pack'. It is hard to account for the resurgence of petrol sniffing which evidently gathered momentum in the late 1960s and early 1970s. At Maningrida, it was said to have started 'like fire...all the tribes came together and sniffed'.

We must assume that in the years in which the practice gathered momentum, recruits began to use the substance because of the collective interest of their age-mates. Young adults in Western society used marijuana in these years in increasing numbers — not that this would have affected Aboriginal people in Australia, but the example illustrates how a particular substance can rapidly gain in popularity. There are two published reports of non-Aborigines sniffing petrol in Australia dating from 1963 in Tasmania and 1967 in Adelaide (Gold 1963; Black 1967).

A series of demographic factors probably also exerted an influence on the spread of sniffing at this time. Altman, for example, notes that the death rate of men in their early twenties in north-central Arnhem Land had decreased by the 1950s, and posits that this was due to the cessation of warfare in the region (Altman 1982, 384). By the 1960s and 1970s the size of youth peer groups had probably increased throughout Arnhem Land and elsewhere as a result of a complex interaction of factors. In addition, the survival rate of infants was increasing from the 1960s (Gray 1985, 25):

> Increases [in fertility rates] during the 1960s...were real for many groups in Government settlements and missions, and may be taken to represent a continuation of recovery from the catastrophic effects of European settlement.

Gray points out some of the pitfalls in assessing fertility rates, pointing out the lack of uniformity in such rates among different regional groups. Whilst recognising the difficulties associated with overall statements because of this regional variation, Gray provides a table showing that in fifteen out of twenty-one named language groups in the Northern Territory, the total fertility rates increased between 1962 and 1971 (1985, 25). In the remaining groups, the fertility rate had increased

THE SPREAD OF THE PRACTICE 143

between 1957 and 1961. Young documents a high rate of population growth at Yuendumu, noting that, although fertility had declined, so had the infant mortality rate between the 1950s and the 1970s (Young 1981, 64). At Ngukurr, there has been a dramatic increase in the survival rate of infants. Nursing staff there observed in 1988 that, whereas the present generation of grandparents would often have had only two surviving offspring, these children (now in their thirties) have up

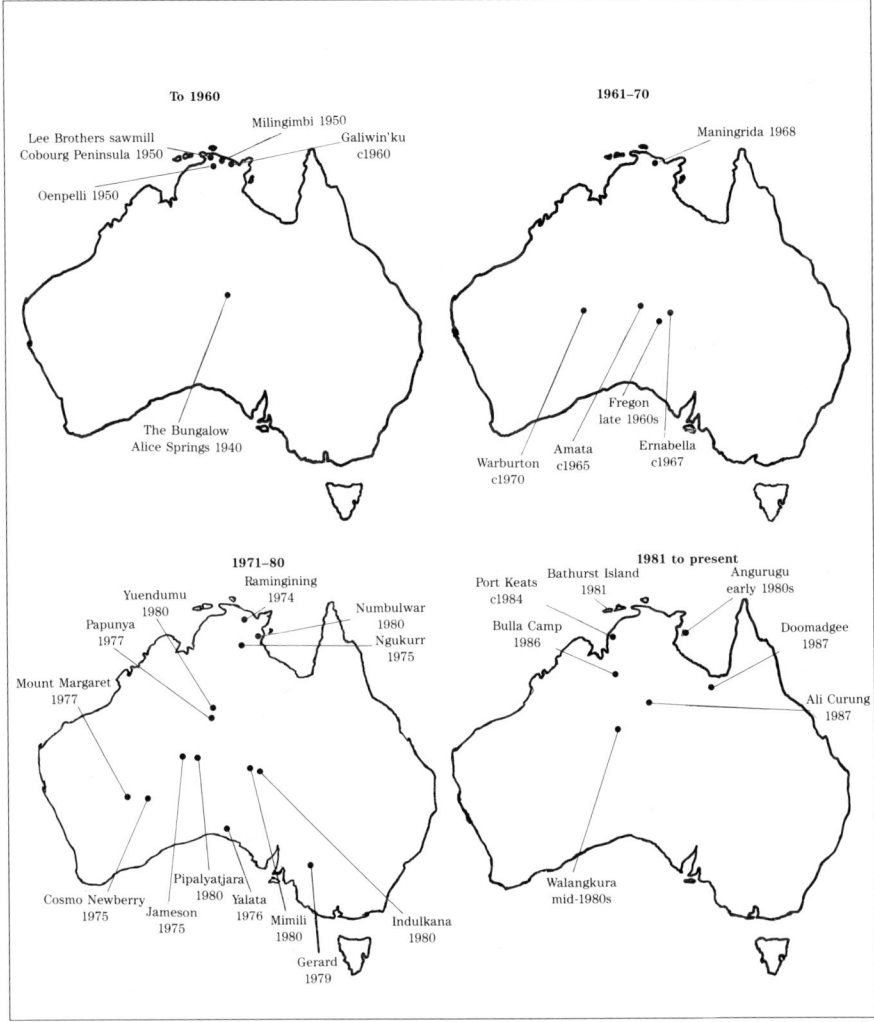

Figure 12: Aboriginal communities reporting their first instance of petrol sniffing up to the present

to thirteen surviving children. By 1980 the youth population (under eighteen years of age) of Maningrida township, for example, constituted 52 per cent of the total population (Altman 1982, 453).

Another factor that influenced the creation of large groups of age-mates was, of course, simply the formation of the settlements themselves, which served to concentrate previously small, dispersed groups. Maningrida, for example, which began its life as a trading post in 1949, was not initially intended to be a permanent settlement, but by 1960 had a population of 480 people from nine different language groups. By 1971 there were over 1,100 Aboriginal people and nearly 200 Europeans (Altman 1982, 7–8). The government policy of assimilation was ratified in 1961, bringing about an intensification of the role of the welfare state in the lives of Aborigines (Altman 1982). Although several missions had been established much earlier than this (Roper River, 1908; Goulburn Island, 1916; Milingimbi, 1925), the settlements became consolidated over this period, and the 'stragglers', who had not previously lived permanently in a settlement, began to adopt this way of life. For example, the Gunwinggu were the last to arrive at Maningrida in the mid-1960s (Altman 1987, 18); the Balamumu arrived at Numbulwar (then Rose River Mission, established in 1952) from Blue Mud Bay in the north, in 1959 (fieldnotes 1985).

McKnight, writing of the people of Mornington Island, discusses the massive increases in population and what he terms 'relational density' (ie the density of others known to an individual by kinship terms). His observations (1986, 157) are pertinent in the wider context as well, for all large communities constitute a 'supercamp':

> The supercamp that the Mornington Islanders live in nowadays is quite different in area, population size, age structure and composition from their traditional camps. The people are aware of these differences. The elderly, in particular, would marvel at the number of children, and claimed that they had never seen so many of them. Occasionally they would ask children who their parents were, in order to be certain about their relationship with them. Complaints about the number of people, the higgledy-piggledy residences and smoke from camp fires, were frequently made. Although I cannot be certain about the exact figures I think it is safe to conclude that, in the past, camps were normally small both in area and population size, and the people who habitually camped together were closely related. Occasionally, larger groups camped together, but only for short periods. It is certain that the whole Lardil tribe never camped together, and no one ever suggested that they did. It would in fact have been economically impossible for them to do so. But nowadays the whole tribe is

> together permanently in one supercamp, along with members of other tribes. As a consequence, not only is the population density high, but so is the relational density.

He goes on to compute the number of relationships between such concentrated groups, so that in a population of 600 people there are 359,400 relationships between those who call each other by a kinship or affinal term. 'This high relational density places a heavy strain on relationships and on the social system as a whole', he observes, because each acknowledges a duty (ideally) to provide help or resources as the occasion demands (McKnight 1986, 158). The strain associated with this density meant that caregivers found it difficult to cope in a situation that can be observed frequently in settlements (McKnight 1986, 152–53):

> Middle-aged mothers had to contend with unruly adolescents who frequently quarrelled and fought with them, and embroiled them in their battles. Some women found it difficult to feed their older children, who were at an age when in the past they would have been contributing to the family larder. In some families, some of the older youths had become what could be regarded as untrustworthy and selfish, for as soon as their mother was out of sight they would raid her meagre hoard of food. In a way they were following traditional practice, for, in the past, food was not normally saved. But it is one thing to act like this when all the family were hunting and gathering, and another when the family live in a village, hunt at weekends, and purchase much of their food supply and modern hunting equipment out of low wages and welfare benefits.

These observations by an anthropologist with twenty years of association with the settlement provide a context within which we can appreciate how population concentrations created ample opportunity for groups of age-mates to congregate in unprecedented numbers. They also illustrate the immense difficulties of controlling the behaviour of others, and even of providing adequate care. Supervision of children, even if it was minimal in earlier times, is virtually impossible in settlements of this size.

The enlargement of the youth population, and the proximity of these youths to each other, brought into being the phenomenon of large associations of age-mates which could form action groups and share social pursuits. The development of schools, particularly boarding schools,[6] for older children also emphasised the groupings of young people, not only because children are schooled together, but live together as boarders. The growth of sports such as football had a similar effect; sporting fixtures mean inter-community events and larger regional meetings (such as Yuendumu Sports and East Arnhem Sports). On all these occasions young people are marshalled and attention is focussed upon them as a group.

These demographic factors are associated with the rise in the prevalence of petrol sniffing in the mid-1960s and 1970s, after the initial experimental incidents which had taken place much earlier. Once more, this analysis has avoided stressing the factors which many other observers assume to be influential: cultural 'breakdown', neglect, and culture clash or the availability of alcohol. Whether there is a historical relationship between access to alcohol and the entrenchment of sniffing is hard to assess realistically, although it would be easy to jump to this conclusion.[7] The right to vote at federal elections was granted to Aborigines in 1962; the right to drink was granted to them (in the Northern Territory) in 1964. As Sansom notes, Aborigines everywhere interpreted the 'citizenship' of 1962 as allowing them to drink and they began to drink openly even before this 'right' had been officially granted (Sansom 1980, 75). This is not to suggest that Aboriginal people had been obediently observing the prohibitive laws applied to them — drinking of beverage alcohols and methylated spirits was indulged in by Aboriginal people who were so inclined, irrespective of the law. But in the 1960s alcohol did not flow freely into the mission settlements of Arnhem Land where petrol sniffing was beginning to flourish, and those who did indulge probably did so in and around Darwin and other centres (see Sansom 1980, 45). It is only comparatively recently that alcohol has been available on demand through deliveries by barge (such as at Maningrida) or through access to licensed clubs (such as at Alyangula on Groote Eylandt and Aboriginal-managed premises like those at Oenpelli and Melville Island).[8]

CENTRAL AUSTRALIA

> Mr Perkins — 'I was petrol sniffing when I was at Bungalow nearly 35 years ago' (Senate Select Committee 1985, 190).

Aboriginal spokesman Charles Perkins's statement that petrol sniffing was known among residents of the institution known as the Bungalow in Alice Springs is not the only evidence of this fact. Another prominent Aborigine, Bob Randall (now a folk singer), said at a 1982 workshop in Alice Springs that he had used petrol there in the 1940s. 'We sniffed using rags', he said, 'talked about dreams and had good fun. It was boredom, alienation, an emotional breakaway. For some it was a habit, for others bravado. I was transferred up north and got alienated from petrol, lost the desire to do it. Some dropped out' (author's notes, Workshop on Petrol Sniffing, see Northern Territory Department of Health 1982).

Although before the war the Bungalow had been a 'half-caste' institution, Harry Giese, the Director of Welfare, made it into an Aboriginal reserve after the war, a depository for people visiting Alice Springs, in an attempt to keep Aborigines out of the town (P Read, personal communication). Like the Lee Brothers sawmill in the north, the Bungalow drew Aborigines of different language groups together. In 1957, for example, at the Bungalow school there were forty-four Arrernte, twenty-three Luritja, six Warlpiri, five Anmatyerre, four Kaytej, two Alyawarra speakers and one Warumungu speaker (Giese 1957).[9] This headcount was undertaken perhaps fifteen years after the reports of petrol sniffing at the Bungalow, as Randall's and Perkins's accounts date it between 1940 and 1942.[10] Even at that time the population at the Bungalow was evidently a mixture of people from different language groups. Whether knowledge of petrol sniffing dispersed from the Bungalow to surrounding regions is unknown, but it seems clear that the experimentation with petrol at the Bungalow never developed into the concentrated use by determined groups of sniffers as occurred twenty-five years later.

As in the north, after these early reports in the central region there was a hiatus until the mid-1960s, when the use of petrol came to prominence, though these new reports did not emanate from the Alice Springs region at all, but further south, on the North-West Reserve, now known as the Pitjantjatjara Lands. Amata (a government settlement established in 1961) and Ernabella (a Presbyterian mission established in 1936) were the two communities where petrol sniffing was first noted in the 1960s.

Bill Edwards, then a missionary at Ernabella, estimates that the practice was first noted there in approximately 1967 and may have been encouraged by the arrival of a thirteen-year-old boy from Amoonguna (just south of Alice Springs). David Hope, previously a superintendent of the government settlement of Amata, recalled that on his arrival in 1968 'petrol sniffing was then actively pursued by groups of pre-initiates — so-called *nynkas* [sic]'. He estimated that it had commenced between 1965 and 1967.[11] Both these observers emphasised the flow of visitors to the area — people from Coober Pedy, Alice Springs, Areyonga, Hermannsberg, Papunya and Warburton.

As already mentioned, by 1970 the practice had escalated to the extent that it was prohibited in the whole of the North-West Reserve (see Hope 1983, 190). Between 1970 and 1980 the first reports of petrol sniffing occurred in a variety of locations associated with these Pitjantjatjara communities (see Figure 12). These communities are interlocked with a network of associations, through language, social organisation, marriage and ceremony (Wallace 1977) — the links which early anthropologists referred to as providing a remarkable unity between Aborigines of the Western Desert bloc, from Kalgoorlie in the west to Port Augusta in the east and to the Northern Territory border region in the north (see Elkin 1931). Pitjantjatjara and Yankunytjatjara speakers have relatives at Yalata and Gerard, and west across the Pitjantjatjara Lands to Warburton in Western Australia (see Figure 13).

Wingellina (on the South Australian–West Australian border), though predominantly Pitjantjatjara-speaking, has links with Ngaanyatjarra speakers in Blackstone, Jameson and Warburton. Warburton people regularly visit Laverton and Kalgoorlie and have ceremonial links with Wiluna. Residents of Cosmo Newberry (previously a United Aborigines Mission cattle station) moved to an outstation of Warburton, Tjirrkali, when it was established in 1982. Warburton region people also have extensive ceremonial links with Coonana (previously

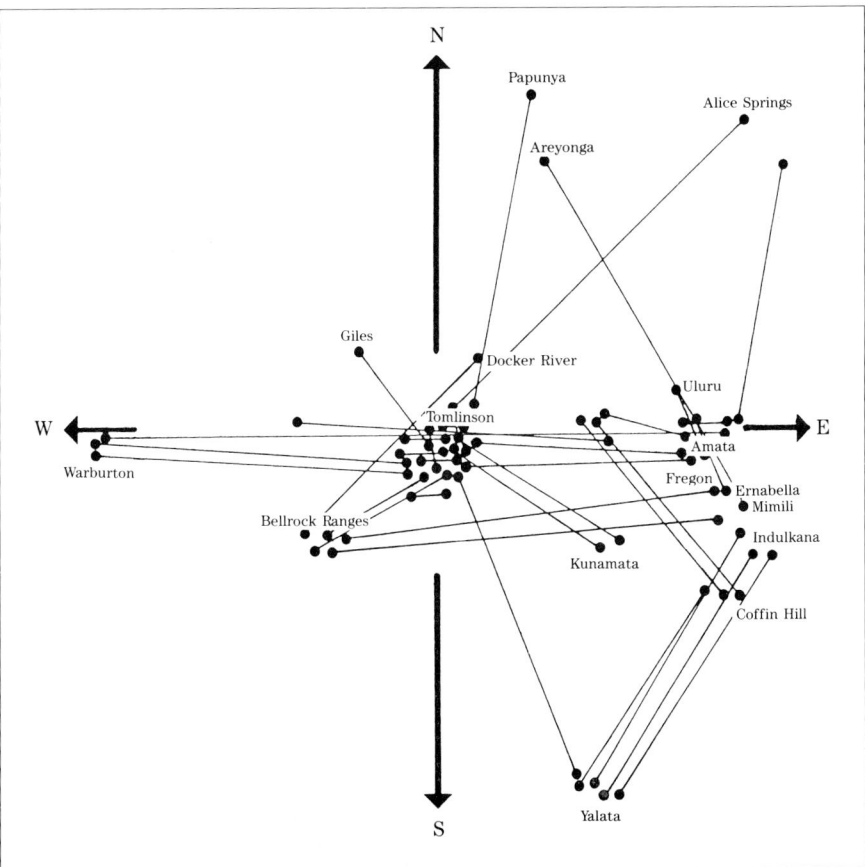

Figure 13: Distribution of marriage alliances in the Pitjantjatjara region (reproduced with kind permission from Hope 1983, 79)

Cundeelee) and with Yalata in South Australia. This is but a brief sketch of the associations which prompt a high level of mobility and residential relocation over hundreds of kilometres in the region. These associations have, inevitably, also meant that familiarity with the practise of sniffing has been communicated and taught. The social proximity of these communities has provided a major impediment to controlling the practice (see Figure 14).

Factors contributing to the increased size of the youth population in this region are similar to those mentioned as relevant in northern Australia — improvements in the rate of infant survival and the concentrations of large populations in settlements and missions. In addition, by the late 1970s private ownership of vehicles by Aboriginal people was becoming more common. Up until this time, not only was vehicle ownership rare (see Hope 1983, 198), but there were many communities without their own petrol pumps. For example, Ernabella's petrol supply consisted of a couple of forty-four-gallon drums of petrol and kerosene with hand pumps until approximately 1967 (B Edwards, personal communication).

In essence, a combination of factors can be blamed for the spread of petrol sniffing, which was so inevitable and so relentless that no-one could interrupt its progress. These factors can be sketched out as follows:

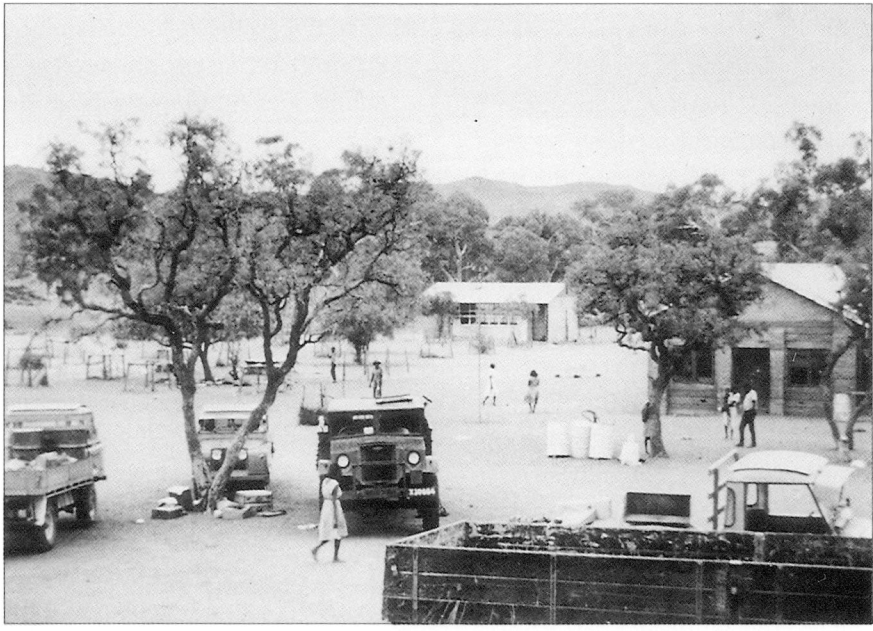

Plate 12: Ernabella central mission compound, 1966, showing full complement of vehicles and a petrol depot consisting of forty-four gallon drums (photograph Bill Edwards)

Historical Forced and voluntary abandonment of small hunter-gatherer group lifestyle; creation of mission and government settlements.

Political Government policies made settlements into institutions; Aborigines became dependent on white systems to solve local problems.

Demographic Lower infant and child mortality; larger groups of age-mates.

Social Creation of teenagers as a social grouping; growth of non-Aboriginal focus on youth; interest in sport and attendance at boarding schools exaggerates teenage group bonding.

Logistical Availability of privately owned vehicles; availability of petrol; mobility facilitated by these two.

Cultural Marriage links and land alliances covering vast distances; contact facilitated by vehicle ownership.

THE PROGRESSION

There are thirty communities for which it has been possible to date the first reported instances of petrol sniffing; 40 per cent reported their first sniffing in the 1980s. Overall, the decades have seen a steady increase in the reported cases from one in the 1940s and three in the 1950s, to five in the 1960s, nine in the 1970s and twelve in the 1980s (see Figure 12). Petrol sniffing has also developed in intensity over the years discussed here, and it is useful to understand this progression as having three stages.

First, there was the initial discovery and use in the 1940s and 1950s. This was purely sporadic and experimental substance use; a small number of individuals dared to experiment with a substance which was not easily obtained.

The second phase commenced after a lull between 1950 and 1960; the actual reasons for the reappearance of sniffing at that time are unknown. This phase lasted through the early 1970s, in which sniffing began to occur in a wide number of locations. In this phase individuals (mostly boys and young men), who are now adults, fathers and uncles of the present generation, used petrol in an experimental way. The sniffing engaged in at this time was not intensive enough to cause large-scale hospitalisation or the development of serious physical sequelae. Many of these individuals rose to political and local prominence, becoming Council members, teachers' aides and even parliamentary representatives. Bill Edwards, commenting on this period, wrote 'those involved were some of the boys from stable families who themselves have become fairly stable members of the communities' (personal communication). Very few of these individuals appear to have experienced any long-term physical effects.

The third phase extends from the mid-1970s to the present, and it was during this period that the practice intensely preoccupied core groups of individuals in some communities. The use of petrol continuously (ie with little or no break) and chronically (ie over a long period of time) has been notable during these years, and has been accompanied by an associated rise in morbidity and death.

The three phases are significant for two reasons. First, the fact that such an intensification has occurred suggests that the users have not adopted self-regulation of their drug use. In other words, the social setting has not provided the context within which the users of today have observed and followed the more moderate using practices of their kin and associates of the previous generation. Instead of this, the development of a continuity of use within the using groups themselves has exerted a greater influence, so that consistent and habitual — rather than occasional — use has become the norm. Second, the pattern of more moderate use (by those who are now the 'older' generation) has served to impede and inhibit direct intervention today. This is because those among the older generation who tried petrol sniffing did not notably suffer physically from the practice, and eventually grew out of it. As Zinberg points out, when users' experiences tells them their drug use is not in itself bad, warnings become unrealistic (1984, 15). Although individuals from this group express 'official' concern about sniffing, their own experience is sufficient to induce a tolerance of the practice and the expectation that it will pass. The matter of tangible physical symptoms associated by Western medicine with the effects of toxic hydrocarbons and organic lead is further complicated by different belief systems which attribute illness and sudden death to other causes. When an individual, who has himself used petrol in the past, loses a son or nephew who has been a chronic petrol sniffer, there is not only a cultural but a psychological imperative to believe that the boy died because someone with malevolent intent adulterated the petrol with battery acid, or because he had been sniffing 'strong' petrol in another community.[12]

Two further issues are clarified if it can be understood that the use of petrol has progressed through these stages and intensified in this way. First, this development helps to explain why petrol sniffing persists today in locations where it has become an established practise over a matter of years of 'accepted' use — up to fifteen years from the development of the second phase. Conversely, it also helps to explain why it is that people in locations where this has not been the case may be relatively successful in curbing its establishment. Second, and more importantly in terms of intervention, it is clear that some determined work is needed to alert the older generation of ex-users to the fact that the patterns of use today are qualitatively and quantitatively different from those of the past. An appreciation of this difference would successfully alleviate the guilt of being a past user and would relieve something of the cognitive dissonance experienced when Council members or parent ex-sniffers find themselves forced by circumstances to penalise sniffers.

PRESENCE AND ABSENCE OF PETROL SNIFFING

The question of why the practice of petrol sniffing is prevalent in some areas and not in others has puzzled several observers and is worth examining. Figure 14 provides a schematic outline of the dissemination of sniffing, and also shows in bare outline its prevalence today. It is no accident that the widest distribution of the practice covers the central and southern regions of the country which are marked by the socio-cultural cohesion of their Aboriginal residents. Although in this central and southern area, language dialects, kin and ceremonial associations are subtly differentiated, a notable unity is nevertheless apparent. People at Gerard in the east and Laverton in the west probably have few direct links, but as a result of historical factors people from Yalata (and earlier from Ooldea Mission on the Trans-Australia railway line) have relatives at Gerard, and also north on the Pitjantjatjara Lands and west to the Kalgoorlie and Warburton areas. The associations between Aboriginal people of Western Desert cultures are thus mediated through key centres of population: Yalata, Amata, Warburton and Coonana. These centres either still experience the chronic use of petrol or have, to varying degrees, curbed its rise among their young residents.

A second network of distribution probably exists in which the communities of Papunya and Yuendumu are pivotal. Papunya is documented to have had petrol sniffers in 1977 (Dalton-Morgan 1978) and I have no earlier reference than this. One of its outstations, Kintore, was established in 1981 and has, since that time, experienced petrol sniffing (Franks 1989). In turn, people from Kintore (Luritja/Warlpiri speakers) have associations with Kiwirrkura (in Western Australia) and Docker River. In its turn, Yuendumu, which has endured sporadic incidents of petrol sniffing since approximately 1980, has residents who travel northwest to Balgo and northeast to Ali Curung. Visitors to Balgo also come from Kintore and Kiwirrkura, both of which experience petrol sniffing from time to time (see Figure 15). However — and here the situation becomes more complex — neither Balgo nor Ali Curung have 'internal' petrol-sniffing groups. If the practice of petrol sniffing is taken up purely as a result of demonstration and subsequent imitation, then how can we explain its non-establishment in communities where residents are in contact with people from communities where sniffing is established?

Both Balgo and Ali Curung are useful illustrations here, for their residents receive visitors from petrol-sniffing communities; their children thus know of the practice. There are several possible interlocking answers to this question. First, for whatever reason, in each of these communities there has been no long-term history of the practice dating from the 1960s or 1970s. This means that the older brothers, uncles, fathers and other kin of today's fifteen to twenty-year-olds were not themselves users of petrol. Because of this, there is no established ambience in which younger people have been consistently exposed to its use. It is important to remember that, in some other communities, a twelve

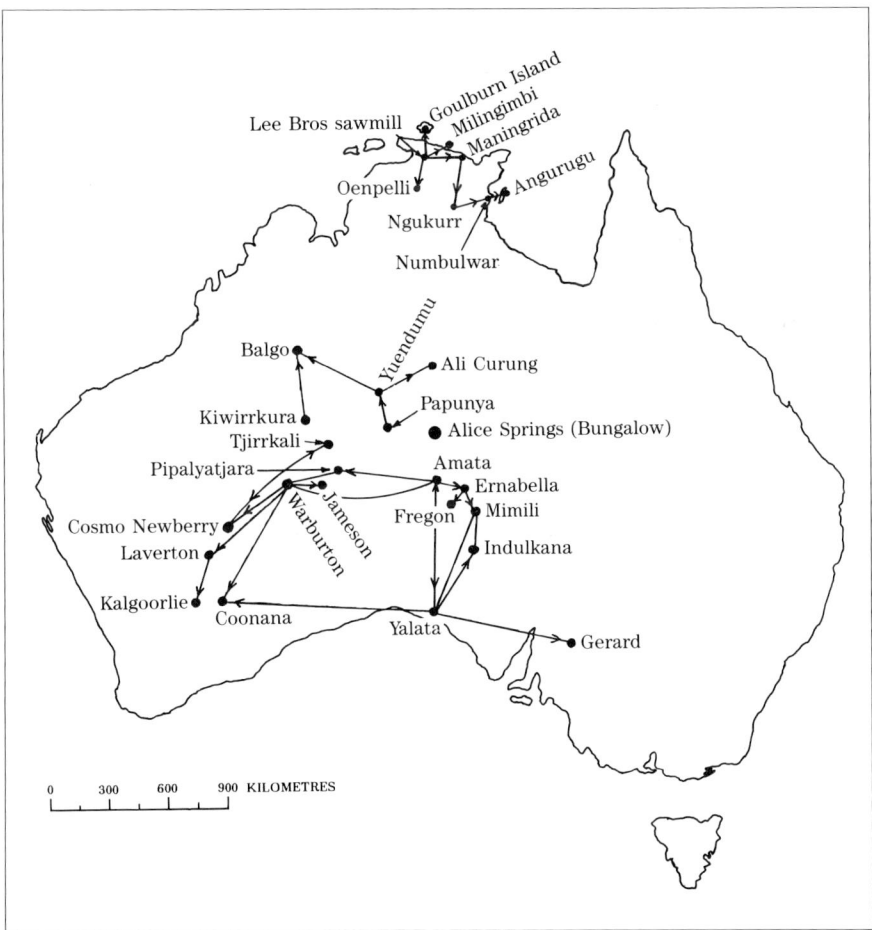

Figure 14: Routes by which petrol sniffing was disseminated throughout Australia

or fourteen-year-old child would have been brought up in an environment where he or she was always exposed to the sniffing behaviour of others, from early childhood. Following from this, if a community contains mature young adults who were themselves sniffers, the population is more likely to be tolerant of the practice — because it has become accepted over time, because those adults (for the most part) seem unaffected physically, and because adults who themselves were sniffers are unlikely to take decisive action about a new generation of sniffers. The absence of an older generation of sniffers is undoubtedly important.

Second, neither Ali Curung nor Balgo have among their present youth population a core group of regular users who could serve to maintain use and recruit new users. This means that when young people from elsewhere who do use petrol arrive for temporary visits, there is no extant using group for them to associate with — they are isolated, and noticeable. Third, in both Balgo and Ali Curung, action was taken decisively and quickly by residents whenever an incoming individual openly used petrol or attempted to recruit others. At Balgo in 1987 when a few young visitors from Kiwirrkura and Kintore were seen walking in the settlement with cans of petrol, they were sent back straight away (S Poirier, personal communication). This observation is reiterated by the late Father AR Peile, long-term resident at Balgo (personal communication): 'There are isolated occurrences of sniffing among young men from Yuendumu and Papunya. These have been kicked out of the community by the people themselves.'[13]

Local perceptions may have had a role here too. Father Piele worked for many years on the Kukatja language, and collected this item on petrol sniffing from a Kukatja speaker:

> Tjitji-lu petrol-pa parntinma; petrol-tjanu parntira
> child petrol smell petrol-from smelling
>
> larlka-rrinpa kaninytjarra kurrunpa dry-pala-rrinpa
> dry-became inside spirit dry-fellow-became
>
> (A child sniffs petrol. As a result of sniffing petrol, the spirit inside [the body] becomes dry, it becomes dry.)

During fieldwork in 1987 at Ali Curung it was said that a boy who had been living at both Willowra and Yuendumu had visited the community in March 1987, and several Warlpiri-speaking children followed his example by sniffing petrol. The sniffers were punished and beaten by older men. Other accounts given by residents were that the practice had come from Alice Springs, or from 'south'; they reiterated that the men had beaten the sniffers and that women had spoken strongly and publicly against the behaviour.[14] The exact details were hard to elicit and despite minor variations between accounts, it appears that action was taken

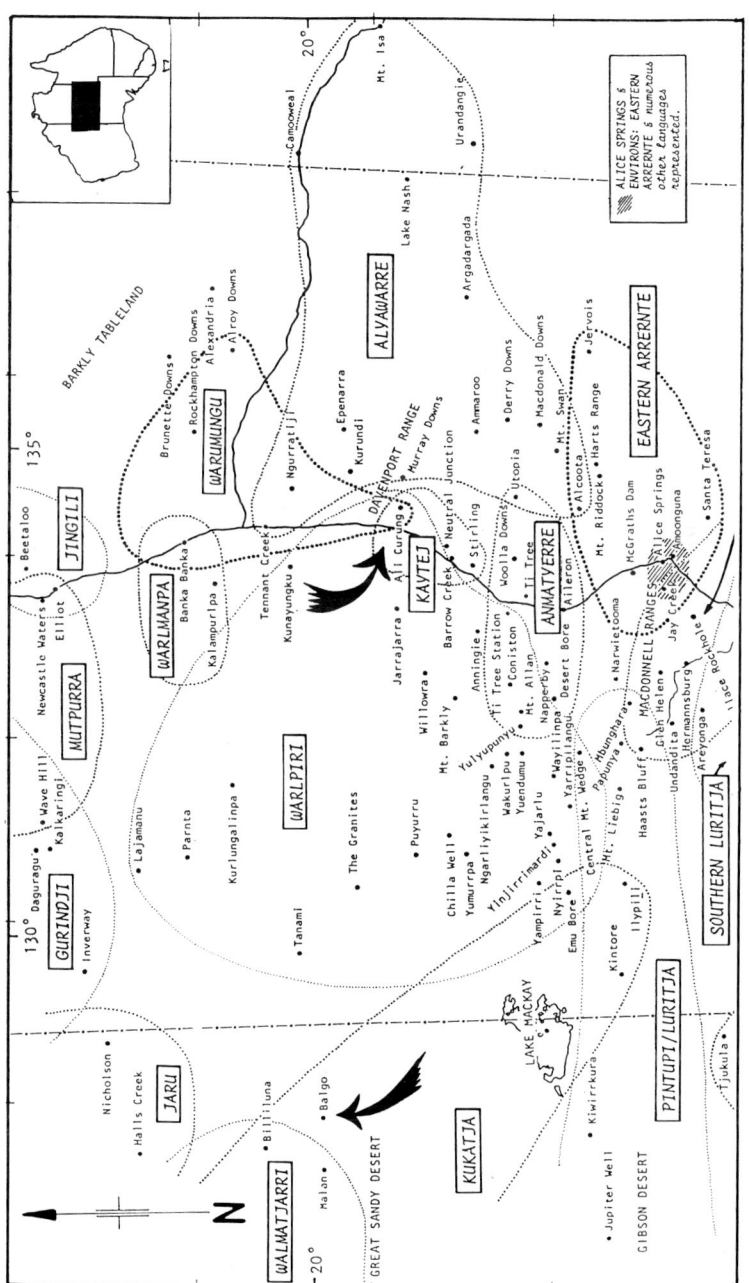

Figure 15: Distribution of Central Australian languages, with reference to Balgo and Ali Curung (reproduced with kind permission of the Institute for Aboriginal Development)

very rapidly to punish those who started to sniff. There is no lack of knowledge about the practice among young people: a young boy voluntarily drew a picture for the clinic nursing sister which featured the words 'Petrol sniffing is BAD! It will spoil your BRAIN. Petrol is for CAR, not for brain!' People at Ali Curung also knew about the use of kava among Arnhem Land residents; they had read about kava in the newspapers during a visit to Darwin.[15]

These communities were 'protected' by the facts that they had no history of use in the form of an older generation who had used petrol; no viable resident group of sniffers; and residents took spontaneous and immediate action when petrol sniffing arrived. There are also geographic and other factors which may have been influential in protecting these communities. Balgo (see Figure 15) is more isolated than many other communities — a glance at the map reveals its position on the edge of the Great Sandy Desert with a sparse population to the south and west. Communities associated with Balgo, such as Mulan and Billiluna, have also taken strong action to prevent sniffing from permeating by banning the sale of petrol. The population centres to the north of Balgo in the Kimberleys have reported little or no petrol sniffing among young members, so the only avenue whereby petrol sniffers visit Balgo is from the south and east. At Ali Curung, the pattern of mobility is diverse and relates to the different language groups who have come to be resident there since 1956, when it began as Warrabri, a government settlement. Warumungu, eastern Warlpiri, Kaytej and Alyawarra speakers now live at Ali Curung. Warlpiri speakers are linked by their associations with Willowra, Lajamanu and Yuendumu; Warumungu speakers with the Tennant Creek area; Kaytej speakers with Neutral Junction; and Alyawarra speakers with Murray Downs and east (see Figure 15). A large contingent from Ali Curung attends the annual Yuendumu Sports. The only avenue of regular contact with petrol-sniffing communities is through the Warlpiri speakers' associations with the west, and southwest to Yuendumu.[16] There is no incidence of petrol sniffing in the surrounding regions to the north, east or south. Indeed, the Barkly Tablelands constitute a large area in which petrol sniffing is entirely absent among Aboriginal people; this is discussed shortly.

Conversely, it could be argued that several features in the development of these communities would have made resistance to petrol sniffing less likely. Both Balgo and Ali Curung people have been institutionalised in earlier years in ways that could seriously affect their parenting behaviour and ability to deal with social problems. Balgo was a Catholic (Pallotine) mission established in 1937, which operated a system of dormitory accommodation and the mass feeding of residents until the 1980s. Although several Catholic priests at Balgo became extremely knowledgeable about the culture and language of their clients (notably Father

Peile), earlier priests there firmly believed that Aborigines were primitive and 'ignorant of their human dignity' (Alroe 1988, 32). Ali Curung, sited insensitively on a sacred Dreaming site in 1955, was virtually a displaced persons camp for Warumungu people, whose land had been invaded by pastoralists and the gold rush of the 1930s, and Warlpiri people who fled after the Coniston killings in 1928. The composition of the present settlement, in which the Warumungu and Warlpiri are still considered by the other language groups to be interlopers on their land, has created and sustained tensions which are manifest in unrest and violence. Access to alcohol at licensed outlets along the Stuart Highway is easy. There was missionary involvement at Ali Curung by the Central Australian Baptists from 1957 and institutionalised mass feeding took place until the late 1960s. Despite these inauspicious histories, both Ali Curung and Balgo have been successful so far in restricting the spread of sniffing among their own young people.

Bulla Camp, near Timber Creek in the Northern Territory, is an example of a small community which took immediate action when petrol sniffing appeared. Jack Little, a man from Bulla who is employed at the Katherine Institute of Health, recounted what happened there in 1987 (personal communication):

> Some young people had stayed at Bulla from Alice Springs, who had learned [sniffing] from Docker River. They were sent back to Alice Springs and told they could come back if they respect the rules. The police had a meeting with the community and told the dangers. They poured the petrol on the ground and threw a match at it and said: 'This is what happens to your brain'. Some kids of about thirteen or fourteen got a flogging from the Council.

All the major settlements (with populations over 200) in Arnhem Land have experienced periods when petrol sniffing has been prevalent among children and young adults. Some no longer have a group of chronic users or have never had a long-term problem. Two communities appear to have been successful in curbing the practice despite several occurrences, notably Ngukurr, and to a lesser extent Umbakumba on Groote Eylandt.

Although Arnhem Land is a network of alliances and associations which link people through marriage, landholding and ceremony, as a general rule these links are more regionalised and localised than in the Western Desert. This regionalisation is associated with a greater diversity of language and clan groups and a tightly knit system of land tenure which means that people are more conscious of boundaries in territory than are Western Desert people. For example, at Numbulwar, and north along the east Arnhem Land coast, twelve territories can be identified, each owned by a different clan; people can define the extent of these areas and they can hold a variety of rights (some shared, some exclusive) over them (fieldwork in 1983–84). Larger socio-cultural blocs exist too: Berndt divided north Arnhem Land into two 'major cultural blocs' differentiated from one another by linguistic units and social organisation, but with 'cultural blurring' on the fringes (Berndt 1976, 145; see Figure 16). As an approximate guide to the associations and mobility of Arnhem Land people, Berndt's classification is still useful. People at Milingimbi tend to be oriented to the eastern communities of Ramingining and Galiwin'ku, while Maningrida residents are oriented to the Oenpelli region and Goulburn Island. The only major communities with few or no instances of petrol sniffing in the west are Croker Island and Milingimbi. As neither was part of this study it is difficult to hypothesise as to why this should be so. Milingimbi children sniffed petrol sporadically in 1974 (I Keen, personal communication) and, as discussed earlier, Milingimbi was one of the first settlements to be associated with the spread of sniffing from the sawmill on Cobourg Peninsula in 1950, as well as being the site of a Royal Australian Air Force base during the Second World War.

In the eastern region of Arnhem Land the two notable exceptions to the chronic or regularly recurring use of petrol are Umbakumba and Ngukurr. Umbakumba is sixty kilometres from the other Aboriginal settlement on Groote Eylandt, Angurugu. While Angurugu has had a strong missionary presence since the first CMS mission at Emerald River in 1921, Umbakumba was administered by the mission for only eight years between 1958 and 1966. The settlement was started in 1938 by Fred Gray, a trepang fisherman and later the caretaker of the flying-boat base there. Gray had an erratic relationship with the missionaries on the other side of the island. He left in 1958, and after a brief period of CMS control, Umbakumba became a government-controlled settlement (Cole 1984). Petrol sniffing did not commence on the island until years after it began at other Arnhem Land settlements, and a long-term resident estimated that it was not until the early 1980s (L Tremlett, personal communication). Tremlett, once the town clerk of Angurugu, recalled that there had been occasional short-lived 'outbreaks' of sniffing. Then some young men from the mainland were sent to the island to attend court for sniffing-related offences and were not returned to their home community. They began sniffing and soon a group of Angurugu young people took up the practice.

Umbakumba people assert that they stopped their children from sniffing using a variety of techniques. Six children were sent away to North East Island (date unknown) to survive there on their own, but they made themselves a raft and one boy drowned after it broke up. 'For this reason', said a Councillor at Angurugu, 'we don't want to do that'. Umbakumba people also made sure that all local vehicles were diesel, and that petrol for outboard motors was locked away.

THE SPREAD OF THE PRACTICE

If children stole petrol the Council members administered a public beating 'in front of everybody's eyes'. This is a type of intervention that can rarely be managed in a community. Umbakumba is protected somewhat by its isolation from other centres of population on Groote Eylandt and its residents do not interact with

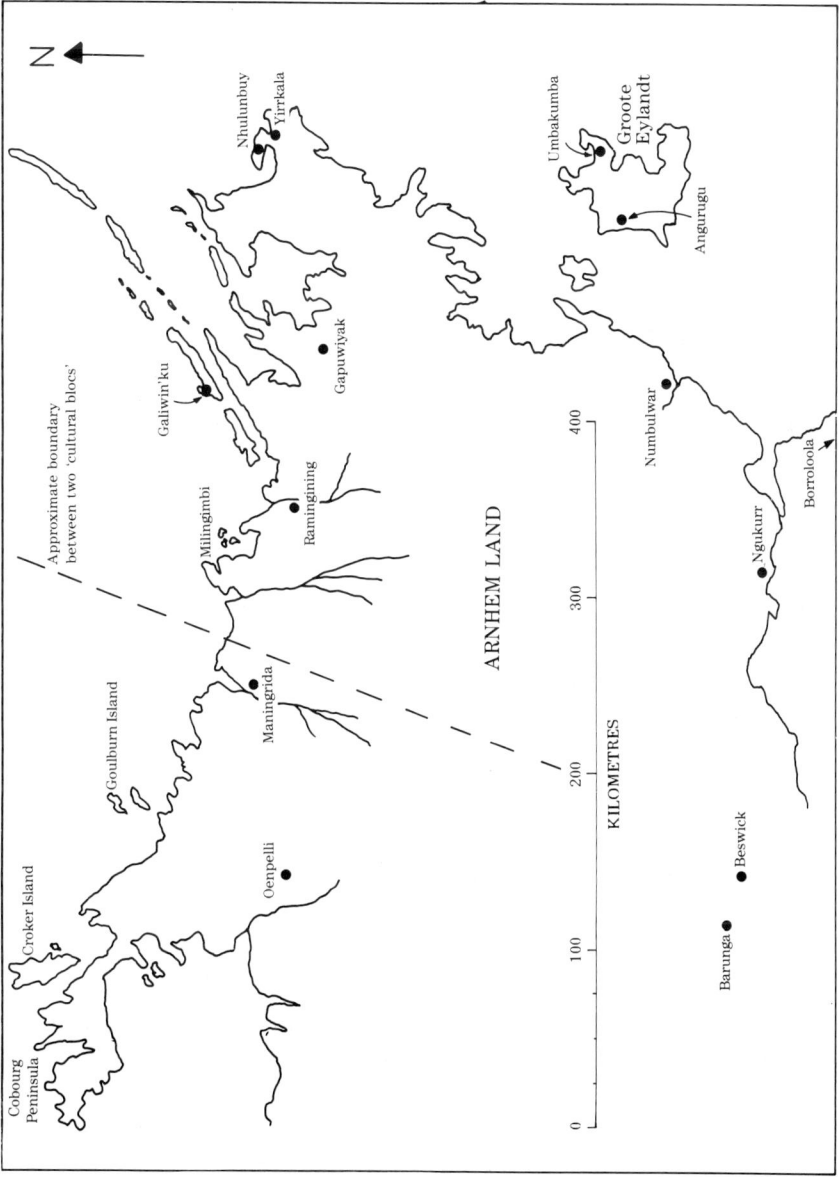

Figure 16: Major Aboriginal communities in or near Arnhem Land (after Berndt, 1976)

mainland communities to the extent that its neighbours on the western side of the island do. It also has no airstrip.

COMMUNITY ACTION

Ngukurr is a community proud of its success in arresting petrol sniffing. Indeed, in November 1986 Walter Rogers, 'President of Yugal Manji Resource Association and Community Leader of Ngukurr', wrote angrily to the Northern Territory *News* after the newspaper (reporting on the Senate Select Committee on Volatile Substance Fumes) listed Ngukurr as being a community where sniffing was practised:

> We have controlled petrol sniffing for more than two years. We have done it without Government assistance and our people are proud of this record. When you say Ngukurr is one of the communities involved in petrol sniffing you make us feel ashamed.

Ngukurr was established as Roper River Mission in 1908 by the CMS, who ran the settlement until 1968 when the government took over the administration. The community is located on land held by Aborigines in freehold title (as is the rest of Arnhem Land) as a result of the Northern Territory Land Rights Act 1976 , and in 1987 it came under Aboriginal administration. Aborigines in the Roper River region had been brutally hunted and shot in the early years of the twentieth century by representatives of a cattle syndicate, who carried out systematic extermination (see Sandefur 1985). The mission attracted the survivors of these atrocities, drawing together people who spoke up to two dozen Aboriginal languages. The CMS instituted a dormitory system and mass feeding; the communal kitchen did not close until 1965. Aborigines worked on large market gardens which produced fresh vegetables. Several women at Ngukurr reminisced about the mission regime:

> Mission had girls' and boys' dormitories and feeding in the cookhouse from Monday to Friday. At weekends people got bush tucker, young girls milked goats, picked up eggs, grew vegies. Before breakfast, jump in the river (really cold). We had to do it because if we don't we get hiding. People lived in camps around mission. School holidays we went out bush with parents. Had a stockyard, young stockmen. People picked their own jobs. Got up early to get firewood...if they miss out work, they got a hiding. Boys used to catch brumbies.[17]

> My people used to be concerned about young people, and tell us where we did wrong. All the old people used to growl at us,

everybody's concern...our parents weren't educated much, but they were strong. When kids did wrong things missionaries and parents punished them straight away.

Old CMS film footage shows white missionary women washing, drying and dressing children, then feeding them; and young people working in the market gardens, and with the cattle herds. These people, now adults in their forties and fifties, run the community with few white staff. With an Aboriginal population of between 600 and 700,[18] there were (in 1987) sixteen white 'staff', including two police officers, who cover a wide area extending south to Nutwood Downs. The local Aboriginalised Anglican church has a strong following, especially among women, who attend nightly Fellowship meetings and have their own choir. Petrol sniffing began at Ngukurr in the mid-1970s[19] and several people I spoke to agreed that this had occurred when a young man from Ngukurr, who had been living at Maningrida, returned to Ngukurr: 'Before that, they didn't know anything'. The Reverend Michael Gumbili described what happened (personal communication):

> One boy came and teach them how to sniff. One boy showed them. E____ and M____ started [early] in the 70s but go slow [here]. Then the boys from N____ started it here [ie again]. The council hunted those boys away. It was young people and young adults, had a group of young people, ten or so. They took them bush to Kangaroo Island [located in the Roper River] they stayed one week — no rifle, no food. The council made an arrangement to live with swag there — no weapons to hunt with — had to look after themselves. Mosquito eat them! Then council went out and collected them. They had a hiding first [before they went away] and another hiding again for few who still sniffed — in public. No help from parents and parents didn't weaken [ie object to punishment]. No relatives took any part for kids. They all pulled one way. The council helped the parents, they take away their [the sniffers] pride. At N____ [another community] the council gives hiding, but parents take part [ie take sides]. No half and half, no half. The whole community must pull — one agreement only.

Aboriginal people from neighbouring communities reiterated the story and there is no reason to disbelieve it. Although this extraordinary example of a coherent action among involved people occurred sometime in the late 1970s, it appears that the firm stance on sniffing has continued to the present. While some of the older women stressed other actions they had taken and downplayed the physical punishment of sniffers, they agreed ultimately that this is what had occurred. One woman described how she had given her thirteen-year-old daughter a 'big hiding' and said, 'I had to cry after that. She [her daughter] said: "Mummy, I'll never sniff that petrol again". Little kids should be looked after and punished so they can learn later on, but you can't really deal with seventeen and eighteen-year-olds.'

The women, many of whom are Christians, said they had given their children who sniffed petrol 'love', they had prayed to the Lord, and given them milk 'to soak up the petrol'. Milk 'make them sober a bit' was another idea offered. Another sanction used at Ngukurr was described by an elderly woman (personal communication):

> I chased my own daughter sniffing — there were married men sniffing [in the 1970s] — 'You make me ashamed!' I said. The women hunted them out. They [sniffers] used to buy petrol from the shop, but we gave the shopkeeper a list of names and said not to give it to them.

That the members of this community should have collectively enacted these sanctions, putting aside the impulse to protect their own children from punishment, is extraordinary. The community is subject to intense political inter-clan disputation (see Bern 1979) over other issues and as mentioned, is composed of a variety of language groups. The early years of the century were marked by a degree of brutality not experienced by Aboriginal groups elsewhere in Arnhem Land, and furthermore, the population was influenced and institutionalised by Anglican missionaries of rigid principles who did not value Aboriginal culture. Bern comments that indigenous controls were curtailed by the mission, and residents were denied the right to apply their own sanctions (1979, 59). His doctoral fieldwork there provoked him to write that (see Thiele 1982, 9):

> The Mission had a strict discipline, which it enforced by a variety of sanctions including fines, removal of privileges, and expulsion....they interfered in all aspects of daily life from personal hygiene to child-rearing.

Thiele documents that, in the early 1970s, the core group (of long-term mission residents) was 'too weak to provide Ngukurr with an active political elite which could enforce its will on the community as a whole' (1982, 16), and that the traditional alliances operated to undermine attempts to establish settlement-wide organisations. The community exhibits all those disadvantages popularly supposed to be the 'cause' of petrol sniffing and yet, in the reported interventions against sniffing, all these disadvantages appear to have been overcome. Several unifying features may have been influential; the first of these is Kriol.

Kriol is a modern language, which developed out of the pidgin English lingua franca of the pastoral frontier; it is the language most commonly used today in Ngukurr. Sandefur, a linguist resident at Ngukurr, associates the origins and growth of Kriol with the disappearance and weakening of different language groups as a result of white incursions, and with the cattle industry. In its earlier form Kriol was already in use by 1908 when the CMS missionaries arrived (Sandefur 1985, 210). Despite opposition from some missionaries and of the anthropological thinking of the time, which saw Kriol as perverted gibberish, missionaries were forced to use it in order to communicate at all. The war years and the employment of Aborigines in the pastoral industry helped to disseminate Kriol, as Aboriginal people moved freely (many for the first time) across the country. Kriol is now proudly used by Ngukurr residents (as it is in many other communities) who produce their own reading materials and booklets in the language. There are now an estimated 15,000 speakers of Kriol across northern Australia (Department of Education, Employment and Training 1989; see Figure 17). Interestingly, the

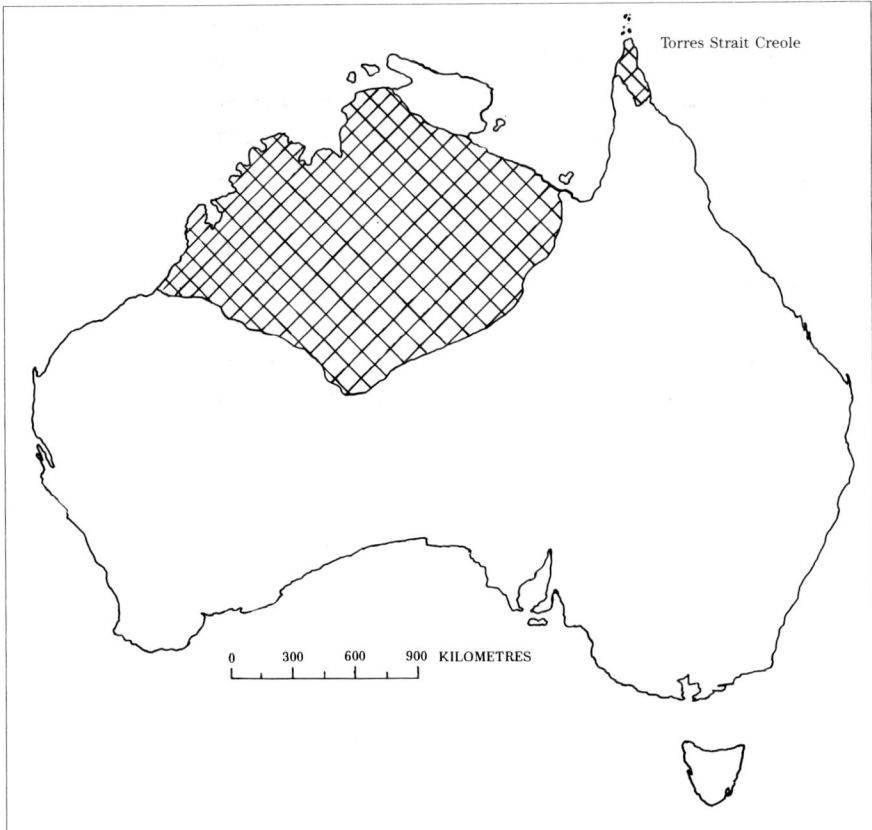

Figure 17: The approximate distribution of Kriol speakers in Australia (this area also contains speakers of at least eight prominent Aboriginal languages)

distribution of Kriol speakers also approximates the regions in which petrol sniffing is rarely, if ever, noted.

Closely associated with Kriol is another factor influential in providing Ngukurr people with a sense of unity and pride (Sandefur 1985, 213):

> After the War...many Ngukurr Aborigines spent months away from their own country on droving trips, travelling east across the Barkly Tablelands deep into Queensland, or south to the railhead at Alice Springs, or west across the Northern Territory to the meatworks at Wyndham. Such droving continued throughout the 1950s and into the 1960s until roads were opened up and modern transport made droving uneconomical.

Today, some of those ex-drovers are instrumental in the growth of cattle and buffalo mustering projects in and around the outstations which have developed from Ngukurr; there are at least eight viable outstations in the region. The men who identify with the cattle industry affect the trappings of the industry: checked shirts, high-heeled boots and big hats. In 1971 Ngukurr men were the first in the Northern Territory to own and operate a cattle station of their own, although this enterprise later collapsed (Thiele 1982). Other enterprising men at Ngukurr have established three Aboriginal companies who hire themselves out to the Council to undertake work: garbage collection and earth-moving; office cleaning; and roadworks and grading.

The third element which may have contributed to the development of a 'corporate' quality among Ngukurr people, has probably been the mission itself, however ironic this may appear. Sandefur writes (1985, 216):

> The current generation is the fifth growing up at Ngukurr. Its lifestyle is now structured in large part by the modern social institutions that were established, structured and, until recently, administered by Europeans.

After the interruption in mission activities brought about by the Second World War, mission policies changed. In the 1950s, long before these practices occurred in most other Aboriginal communities administered by either government or a mission, Ngukurr established a station Council with equal numbers of Aborigines and staff members in an early — though not particularly successful — attempt to bring about local internal control. The CMS paid 'pocket money' to Aboriginal workers from 1951, and later full wages: this seems patronising today, but it was unusual at that time for Aborigines on settlements to deal in cash rather than rations and other material goods. Also in 1951, the school employed up to eight Aboriginal monitors who supervised classes once work had been set (Sandefur

1985, 214). In 1987 the Ngukurr school had an Aboriginal principal, nine Aboriginal teachers and support staff and only three non-Aboriginal teachers.

While the CMS had discouraged and disapproved of traditional religious practices, it was unsuccessful in attempts to undermine them. The CMS monthly report for March 1970, for example, noted that a 'Yabadurrawa corroboree [sic] [had] been going on for six months...nearly every man involved...had a real effect on church attendance and personal loyalties'. The report goes on to note that very few men had attended church on Good Friday as they had been 'painting up' for their ceremony (Bern 1979). Today Ngukurr has a devoted Christian following. Several ex-missionaries who served the CMS there maintain contact visits with the community, attending annual Bible Camps which are entirely Aboriginal-organised. Overall, for a variety of reasons, the mission seems not to have brought about or reinforced the sense of Aboriginal dependence on resources provided by whites often noticeable in other areas. There is no expectation among Ngukurr people that the whites are there to make their decisions or solve local problems. Instead, the institutionalising influence of the mission appears to have instilled the idea that the population should submit itself to the decision-making powers of a representative (Aboriginal) body. The councils of the last few years have taken on this role, and the population has acquiesced, at least to the extent that the actions against petrol sniffers were allowed and were not undermined by family influence or loyalties. The politically aware Council members view themselves as having the responsibility for taking decisions. For example, after attending a community meeting of vague parameters instigated by visiting health officials, at which 'community opinion' was sought, a Council member observed, 'If they waited for community opinion they'd have a hundred different ones. They should have had an executive council meeting — we have to pull the community along behind us!' This is a very different state of affairs from that noted by Bern and Thiele in the early 1970s.

It must be said that Ngukurr people have internalised many of the values and principles espoused by the missionaries. The missionaries gave 'hidings' to their charges, and in turn their charges now give hidings to their own children. There is what Bern called a core group of Aborigines at Ngukurr who are permanently resident there and were closely associated with the CMS. They had higher European education levels, lived in better houses, and were less constrained by traditional marriage rules than others (Thiele 1982, 15). These people became dominant in local politics and on the early station Council. Their shared experiences of the early days, and shared Christian beliefs, as well as (paradoxically) a common association with two major ritual cults, have melded a large section of the community into a solidary group (see Thiele 1982, 15). It was undoubtedly these people, comprising three main family groupings, who were pivotal in the Council actions taken against sniffers.

Ngukurr stands as an example of a community which has successfully inhibited petrol sniffing. Aboriginal people there were willing and pleased to discuss the issue. However, it is important to point out that physical punishment alone has been tried and found unsuccessful in other cases. The Ngukurr experience is not presented as a case study promoting the use of physical punishment, and it is likely that the shared determination of adult residents not to tolerate the practice was a key factor in their success in dealing with sniffers. Despite many other splits and the intensity of local political activity, 'all pulled one way' on that particular issue.

NOTES

1. In 1981, the Chief Minister of the Northern Territory told the Legislative Assembly that sniffing had begun when the Royal Australian Air Force (RAAF) first brought in high octane fuel (Adelaide *Advertiser* 28 August 1981). Roger Sigston (ex-resident of Milingimbi) reported that he had been told by local Aborigines that RAAF men had sniffed petrol (personal communication).

2. Professor Powell kindly gave me access to some of his document collection (housed in his office at the University College of the Northern Territory, Darwin).

3. This document was brought to my attention by the remarkable memory of Richard Baker, to whom I am indebted.

4. Thanks to Jon Altman, Greg Jarvis, Trish Joy and Luke Taylor for their help in tracing these individuals.

5. A resident of Bathurst Island (where there is now no reported petrol sniffing) said 'We used to know about it before' (J Devitt, personal communication).

6. Dupama College (now closed) in Gove is thought by some observers to have facilitated the spread of knowledge about sniffing in the 1970s. Considerable numbers of Northern Territory Aboriginal children attend boarding high schools in Queensland, such as Slade College.

7. For example, a beer club opened at Maningrida in 1969 (Altman 1987, 12) around the time when sniffing was first reported.

8. Northern Territory Aboriginal communities (as at 1988) operate nine licensed clubs with a variety of regimes of control, under the Northern Territory Racing, Gaming and Liquor Commission.

9. I have changed Giese's original orthography to the modern orthography.

10. Perkins was born at the Bungalow, the Telegraph Station reserve, in 1936 or 1937 of 'Arrente, Kalkadoon, Pitjantjatjara and Irish descent', and lived in the area until he was 'about ten' (Perkins 1975, 17).

11. Correspondence with David Hope, 25 July 1989 and Reverend Bill Edwards, 31 August 1989.

12. Both of these examples are from my field notes.

13. In June 1991, however, it was reported that some Balgo residents had commenced sniffing (Dr H Saddler, Dr S Cane, personal communication).

14. Another version would have it that Ali Curung children had gone to Papunya and Areyonga and that 'they [people at those places] learnt them how to sniff'; however, one woman Council member believed that there was no sniffing in 1987 at Ali Curung because the recreation hall was open every night, with regular discos, games and videos. There are two local bands, one rock and one country and western.

15. Knowledge of kava had also come from meeting Arnhem Land people at Batchelor College (an Aboriginal teachers' college). Ali Curung people referred to kava as 'milk beer'.

16. A researcher at Ali Curung observed in 1988 that there were very few privately owned vehicles in the community; vehicles are impounded if anyone is caught carrying alcohol in them. This means that mobility is somewhat restricted (G Stotz, personal communication).

17. Keith Hart, a CMS member, was an experienced stockman who worked with the young men; brumbies are wild horses.

18. The Australian Bureau of Statistics Census (1986) records 292 males, 333 females and a total of 625. Clinic records at September 1987 state a population of 367 males, 374 females and a total of 741.

19. John Bern, who undertook his doctoral fieldwork there in 1970–71, confirmed there was no sniffing during those years.

CHAPTER

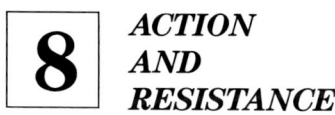

8 ACTION AND RESISTANCE

In order to gain some overall understanding of why it is that this drug abuse, while touching a large number of communities briefly, becomes entrenched in some, we need to examine socio-cultural and attitudinal factors, as well as assessing the level of direct action taken in communities. It is also helpful to take a broad view of the regions in which petrol sniffing is not a regularly used substance. This chapter brings together some of the themes touched upon so far, and then examines factors which seem to characterise communities where inhalant use is not practised.

SOCIAL MEANINGS

Perceptions of the effect of substances (in the widest sense of that term) on an individual's nature are obviously important mediating factors in a society's engagement with such substances. Western populations have particular understandings of drug substances in which the concept of addiction is still widely held to be of principal importance — the notion that the subject submits to a drug agent. Consequently there is a perception that drugs can alter a user's 'nature' on a permanent basis. Drug use is also commonly bound up with perceptions of self-gratification and hedonism, which can lead to the adoption of a moralising stance from which drug use is viewed by the wider public.

Unlike our society, which has a penchant for labelling the deviant or ill among our number, the Aboriginal people with whom I worked were less willing to typify and stigmatise others in this way. Among southern Pitjantjatjara people in South Australia, for example, only a few individuals known to be seriously mentally or physically disordered were perceived to be permanently affected by their disability, and social constructions had been developed which 'explained' why they had become so. These included explanations associated with transgressions of Aboriginal Law or with incidents (usually a wrongdoing or error) that had occurred in the remembered past. However, individuals who became disordered after ingesting substances such as alcohol or petrol were, on the whole, not stigmatised and were perceived to be only temporarily changed. These understandings of the effects of drugs are similar to those of Pacific Islanders who, according to Lindstrom (1987, 11), 'do not expect drug use to bring about permanent transformation in the consumer...they are not concerned to worry about changes in a person's 'nature' brought about by heavy use or abuse of drugs'.

It is true that the mood-altering effect of drug substances on the person occurs more or less immediately and, moreover, wears off (Lindstrom 1987).

Individuals (being users of alcohol or petrol) then, to a greater or lesser extent, resume their non-intoxicated personas. This assessment was reinforced by my experiences in the field which showed me that users of petrol, once back with their home or hearth group, were treated quite normally and resumed day-to-day activities. In an east Arnhem Land community, I observed a young married man in his early twenties who used petrol regularly and had assumed the full trappings of a tough Rambo figure. After several periods in gaol, his body muscles were well-developed from weightlifting practice. He wore a punk style 'Mr T' haircut (with one ridge of hair and shaved sides) and, when sniffing with the other young men, wore elaborately slashed denim jeans, army boots and singlet. One Sunday morning I was surprised to see him without his large cassette player and other distinguishing attire, wearing shorts and a shirt — the normal clothing adopted by men in that region. He was taking a calm early morning stroll with his wife, gently holding his young infant in his arms.

Discussing alcohol use in Papua New Guinea, Marie Reay proposes that the people she studied had a special aptitude for role playing, enabling them to switch from being one person at one moment to quite another the next moment. She provides examples: the role of the bereaved mourner who must be seen to express grief in demonstrable ways; the observation and relinquishing of taboos; and the regular drinker who suddenly assumes the identity of a non-drinker once resolved to abstain (Reay 1982, 167–68). Such a proposition is relevant, for example, when considering whether there is an indigenous conception of 'addiction' — a permanent 'component of the soul' (Kohn 1987, 36). Certainly Aboriginal people refer to petrol sniffers as being unable to stop and say that 'they get used to it' which could be interpreted as a form of habituation. Such observations also communicate the despairing attitude evinced by so many Aborigines in which such rationalisations serve to mask non-intervention. On the other hand, in communities where sniffing has been common over many years, the experience of residents tells them that users do stop sniffing — everyone knows of individuals who were once 'sniffers'. They stop without any outside intervention in most cases. In a central Arnhem Land community, I found that over a period of three years, at least 34 per cent of petrol sniffers had given up the practice.

If drug or alcohol use, and the social life that accompanies it, is viewed as being part of a role adopted at one period of life, surely the notion of addiction fails to account for what occurs? An unknown number of Aboriginal people spontaneously give up drinking and encounter others who have done so (see Laurie and McGrath 1985, 88). The reality of these instances cuts across the notion of addiction for Aboriginal people. It is more common for substance use to be perceived as a 'stage' — individuals engage with petrol, or alcohol, at different times in their lives. A woman at a South Australian community once told me that she had scolded her son for 'still' sniffing petrol when he was old enough to drink alcohol (Brady 1985a). Individuals also resort to drug use on occasions when feeling grief or expressing anger. In another useful observation, Reay notes that aspects of traditional life and belief systems can contribute to the ease or difficulty with which people abstain from drug substances. She suggests (1982, 166):

> People with a tradition of obeying taboos on enjoyable food and activities — sometimes for long periods — should be better able to relinquish alcohol than those in a laissez-faire society with no strong taboos or in which these apply only in certain sectors of society from which it is possible to escape.

This is an interesting idea which could have value in intervention or educational strategies. Food prohibitions or restrictions are widespread among Aboriginal populations in several regions of Australia and are observed to varying degrees. In central Arnhem Land, for example, pregnant women are subject to a variety of food restrictions which are intended to protect the unborn child. Menstruating girls and boys undergoing circumcision should ideally observe certain rules. Pitjantjatjara people in South Australia also assert that they have food restrictions for pregnant women (particularly on large or spiky animals), as do numerous other language groups. Mourning, too, can entail the eschewing of certain favoured food items. As Reay suggests, such restrictions indicate that 'giving up' — if only for a short period — is a part of the cultural milieu and has socially accepted meaning.

Another important influence on how people react to and perceive drug use is related to their expectations of how people behave when they have ingested/inhaled the substance. I have discussed elsewhere the attitudes to drunken comportment among Australian Western Desert people, in which it is accepted that drunken people are not 'themselves' and so their excesses are allowed and excused (Brady and Palmer 1984). During my research I found that some Aboriginal people attributed extraordinary powers to intoxicated petrol sniffers, believing that they had X-ray vision and that they 'had eyes in the backs of their heads'. A sniffer described his experience as being 'hot in the brains'. Women in one Western Desert community thought that 'they can run faster because that juice [petrol] helping them — same like motor car. They act fast'. Aboriginal observers also likened the petrol high to drunkenness, and considered the behaviours to be out of control: 'They break in when drunk from that petrol; make a mess when somebody away, do toilet on it. Hit the shop, clinic, run amuck. They swear in Wongai side [Aboriginal language] and English'.

These socially derived meanings and expectations have a profound influence on how community members deal with these drug takers. It seems, judging by some of these comments, that adults are somewhat in awe of sniffers who are thought to have supernatural powers. Those who liken the intoxication of sniffers to that of the inebriated are likely to believe that, like drinkers, sniffers are beyond control and reason and therefore not responsible for their actions. This brings about a situation in which the drug takers themselves are not blamed for their actions, for they are perceived to be acting involuntarily.

A common expression used in Pitjantjatjara and many other Aboriginal communities is to say that petrol sniffers 'can't listen' (ie will not, or are unable to listen or understand). Sniffers are said to have 'no ears' — for many desert Aboriginal peoples, the ears are metaphorically the organs of understanding and reasoning. A sniffer is 'without ears' and therefore without comprehension (see Brady 1985a, 28). If an individual has no comprehension of the waywardness of his or her actions (as is the case of a sniffer 'without ears') then it is considered to be pointless to try to chastise or reason with that person. A child who has no ears, and therefore lacks understanding and reason, is conceived as being 'wild' and beyond control. The ears are also associated with the emotions of concern and worry, so that an individual telling of her preoccupation and worry about some relatives expressed this non-verbally by cupping her hand to her ear as if listening. A person who cannot 'hear' because of the disordering effects of petrol fumes is also unable to worry or be concerned about their actions. This has a profound influence on the way in which kin relate to each other, for relatedness is expressed through concern, worry and compassion, as Fred Myers has explained (Myers 1986). The existence of this complex of beliefs has served to undermine serious attempts to confront petrol sniffers.

The belief that certain ingested substances can act upon individuals, making them 'different' and unable to control themselves, may also mediate responses to those who ingest mood-altering drugs. For example, in parts of Australia certain substances may be utilised by Aboriginal people in order to procure a desired lover, or to achieve success in some other sphere (such as gambling). In the Kimberley region objects associated with 'love magic' (referred to as *tjirri*) include coloured rocks and powders, small pieces of wood and bone (Akerman and Bindon 1986). Although love magic items can be used in a variety of ways (rubbed onto the hands or body and so on), the most direct method of administration is to add the substance to a cigarette or to a drink which is to be smoked or drunk by the desired partner. Once this is done, that person will be irresistibly drawn to the person who administered the substance. Discussing sorcery and love magic among an island population of Papua New Guinea, Lepowsky (1982, 331) draws a parallel with perceptions of the influence of alcohol:

> The people of...are well known...for the potency of their magic and their sorcery. The islanders are therefore accustomed to the idea that a particular substance may be imbued with the power to take away one's will or make one do the bidding of others.

In Aboriginal Australia, then, it is also a tradition (in some regions at least) for people to lose control, and become not responsible for their actions after they have ingested certain substances. These local understandings may also influence attitudes towards petrol or alcohol-induced comportment. If people so affected are not deemed to be responsible for their actions, it is simply less likely that anyone would be willing to criticise or curtail their activities.

These social meanings associated with sniffing result in an overall perception that the individual is not responsible for his or her actions and this tends to reinforce an externalisation of blame which can have political implications. This externalisation of causality and of the responsibility for sniffing is prevalent among Aboriginal communities. It is notable that people frequently do not 'blame' the toxicity of the petrol itself for the illness and death, and thus by implication avoid accepting that an individual has brought about his or her own death through chronic use of the substance. Blame is levelled at other supposed poisons that have entered the petrol (such as battery acid), or at other communities or individuals who are thought to be implicated in a death. It is also notable that in each community petrol sniffing was said to have originated from somewhere else, to the extent that the same communities blame each other's youth for teaching their own how to sniff. The parents of petrol-sniffing children denied that their own children sniffed, or said that, if they did, it was because others persuaded them.

Externalising blame enables community members to complain that the teachers/nursing sisters/local petrol-sniffing team/government are not doing their jobs properly. If there is a government-funded program in operation involving, for example, visiting teams of people, the externalising of blame enables residents to allocate the responsibility for subsequent deaths to the 'failure' of the program, that is, to individuals from outside the community. Such thinking is not only usually wrong, it is also unhelpful. If Aboriginal people in some areas are still not convinced that petrol is a highly toxic substance when continuously inhaled, then there has been a serious breakdown in communication over the last thirty years. There is little doubt that government agencies were slow to respond to the intensified use of petrol which became manifest in the 1970s.[1]

SOCIAL ACTIONS

In order to deal with the problem of petrol sniffing, a rapprochement must occur between the socio-cultural understandings of Aboriginal people and practical intervention, and in some instances such a rapprochement has taken place. I have described how some communities have agreed by consensus not to tolerate the use of petrol in their midst. They have set aside family loyalties and adapted aspects of loyalty and the requirement to support kin which have enabled sanctions to be taken against the practice by the whole community and/or its Council. The use of physical punishment was thought to be successful by residents in some communities, although the success was probably due to the fact that the community acted cohesively rather than to the means chosen to implement this.

In some settlements (such as Balgo and Ali Curung) and other smaller decentralised groups (such as Punmu in the Rudall River region of Western Australia), the occasional arrival of a petrol sniffer immediately produced group sanctions in which kin-based sentiment was set aside. In many other settlements, however, the active roles taken by individuals to protect their younger kin and to deflect responsibility have meant that corporate action has proved unworkable. Unless people can address these problems frankly it is probably counterproductive for communities to persist in strategies which elicit these defensive responses. Attempts to raise self-esteem and pride among a particular group can contribute to an atmosphere in which differences may be set aside.[2] Other interventions stress the role of the family. The family-based approach is pursued by HALT, which has worked in several Central Australian communities (see Franks 1989; Lowe 1988). HALT has adopted the role of counselling individuals who were related to petrol sniffers 'to take up their traditional parenting roles, which many had abandoned under the stress of the problem' (Franks 1989, 17). Although the team also holds meetings 'to increase broad community cohesion and diminish the isolation...of the family groups', its approach is focussed on caregivers, not on the community as a whole. One of the more effective approaches to petrol sniffing among some native American populations has been intense parental involvement in monitored alternative activities, together with parent 'patrols' so that young people simply could not escape adult observation (Oetting et al 1989, 15).

For very practical reasons, on decentralised outstations sniffing does not usually occur even if their residents include those who usually sniff elsewhere; the reasons are partially related to population and relation density. Life is less subject to interpersonal strain in a smaller group. Sniffing activities are minimised, too, because closer supervision is possible and large groups of age-mates are not usually present. However, outstations are not a panacea for petrol sniffing — some groups do not have freehold title to their land, lack the resources and mobility necessary for establishing outstations, or are politically entrenched in the home settlement. Young men used to speeding around the settlements in cars or on motorbikes, listening to rock music and identifying with teenage gangs, are likely to find the pace of life slow on an outstation. There may be complex matters of land tenure and jurisdiction over others to be considered. In Arnhem Land, for example, the process of identifying land owned by different groups is intricate and ownership rights can be exclusive (rather than inclusive), so that the selection of 'clients' for so-called rehabilitation at an outstation can be limited by various affiliations.

For reasons mentioned earlier, the disease model that is used to explain and treat substance abuse does not always appear to fit closely with Aboriginal perceptions, nor with Aboriginal experience (in which substantial numbers of individuals undergo spontaneous remission from their substance abuse). Nevertheless, the disease model provides the thrust behind the interventions by CAAPS (Council for Aboriginal Alcohol Program Services), an interdenominational Christian church-based program in the Northern Territory. CAAPS is, in fact, the only agency offering residential programs for Aboriginal petrol sniffers (and alcohol users), which provide a hiatus between gaol or hospitalisation and return to home communities. The Aboriginal communities serviced by CAAPS include the west Top End (Bathurst Island to Port Keats); West Arnhem (from Croker Island to Jabiru); east Arnhem (from Maningrida to Yirrkala) and southeast Arnhem (from Ngukurr to Groote Eylandt). The Catholic, Uniting and Anglican churches are associated with the group. The model put forward by CAAPS (nd) makes use of

> concepts developed through the Hazleden and Johnson Institute, Minnesota, USA; Holyoake Institute, Perth, Australia; Alcoholics Anonymous and Al Anon...chemical-dependency is a progressive disease...[that] can be arrested but not cured...[and which] is characterised by highly developed patterns of denial and delusion in both the dependant and those close to him or her.

This has become known colloquially as 'co-dependency'. CAAPS family workers reside in several communities and work directly with users (of petrol, alcohol and kava) and with groups of 'co-dependents' — the relatives of users. The core of their approach is 'tough love', which is based on the idea that (CAAPS nd)

> people who have that feelings sickness will only look for or accept help to stop drinking or sniffing when they are hurting badly from their drinking or sniffing. That will only happen when those who love that person stop caretaking and let the person take the full pain from their drinking or sniffing. Only then will the drinker or sniffer start to know how bad things *really* are.

The approach is simple, and goes directly to the heart of the substance abuse problem, tackling the feelings of guilt and helplessness experienced by the relatives of users. However, there are substantial drawbacks associated with applying these methods to Aboriginal people. Aboriginal family relationships are based on the giving and receiving of help, resources and care. While these relationships and exchanges are abused, inevitably, by categories of individuals (particularly drinkers), these aspects of relatedness are ideals to which all Aboriginal people must aspire. As O'Connor (1988, 119) notes:

> Although the Co-dependents programme claims to be adapted to suit Aboriginal people, grave doubts surround its applicability to traditional people. In that it advises against the fulfilling of traditional kin responsibilities at times, it could be seen as counter-cultural.

The development and use of the term 'co-dependency' has been thoroughly and critically analysed by Lisansky-Gomberg (1989). Despite these criticisms, it is timely for Aboriginal people to look more closely at the consequences of unconditional support for alcohol abusers who exploit kin. Merv Gibson has already questioned this distortion of the ethic of generosity (Gibson 1987). With petrol sniffers (rather than alcohol users) perhaps this is more difficult. Some, though not all, sniffers are young people still dependent on their families for food and housing. Perhaps the main drawbacks with the CAAPS approach are its adherence to the disease model and its Christian religious orientation. Both detract from its appeal to certain sections of the Aboriginal population. Many youths who sniff petrol are already decisively opposed to the Christian elements within their own communities, going out of their way to deride and mock the Fellowship sessions which often dominate the evenings' events. If the only treatment programs to which they are exposed also espouse the Christian ethic, there is a danger of reinforcing a polarity between users as anti-Christian and non-users being identified with Christians and 'missionaries'.

Only once during the course of my field research did I encounter a Council chairman who called a meeting with the youth of his community to find out what they wanted or needed, in a bid to counteract petrol sniffing. This was in an east Arnhem Land community. The chairman described the meeting (personal communication):

> We had a meeting with the young people on the oval. 'What are you really interested in? If you're interested in sport and recreation, I need your help to get it started' [I said]. They said the Council was not interested in their life, just in the community, in houses. 'Council only supports the people, not the young people.' I said, 'Now I'm the chairman, I'm interested in your life and the community. I need you to give me time because of this.' They want to feel happy and wanted. The Council has given the boys the old workshop and the kids helped to clean it up.

Council chairpersons naturally find it hard to devote attention to the needs of youth while they are dealing with a host of other issues. As this man said: 'The community give you that load, and you've got to work your way out'. There is often little real support either from other Council members, or from the community as a whole (Council chairman, east Arnhem Land, personal communication):

> At X they all pull together, all one mob; they support council. Here, I have to do everything and community don't do their part. Two council members from each clan, and they've supposed to talk to parents about sniffing. I've tried three times to talk about sniffing at community meetings and it never happens.

He complained that people 'only think of pay' — and that there is no commitment to voluntary work. Nevertheless, this man started a fund to buy recreation equipment for the young people. He walked around the settlement card games with a donation tin and persuaded gamblers to put money in for sports and recreation, collecting $300. He applied to different government departments and the Aboriginal Benefits Trust Account for funds, finally succeeding after long and painful delays. Six months later he wrote (personal communication):

> My plans for recreation is working very strongly. We had funds to buy some stuff like softball equipment, footy, basketball and volley ball. We have been getting prices for other equipments and should be getting them on the next barge…now everyday people from all ages play softball, footy, basketball. The petrol sniffing have stopped after you left, because the people have seen what happen to some of our boys they got sick…they went into hospital…and now they're back they've seen a big move have been done towards recreation.

A games room was started, equipped with weightlifting gear, pool and darts. The chairman announced that adults could use the community truck 'any time' to take the young people out bush. He wrote to the magistrate asking him not to send young offenders to gaol but to send them for community work somewhere else. This example shows that one person's energy directed to youth issues can transform a situation, but the communities on the whole are dominated by adult concerns, adult priorities and adult enterprises. The distribution of resources and money is undertaken by adults, who tend to favour their own projects. For example, in one east Arnhem community, which received over $1 million in royalties from a mining venture in 1988, only $35,000 was earmarked for sport and recreation, and most of that was taken up by the salary of a recreation officer. In another example, among communities in South Australia who received a $500,000 grant (partly as compensation for past damage to their environments and the consequent dislocation of the people from their lands), the decision was made to spend this on building a road to link their communities to others several hundred kilometres away. This decision benefits primarily older men, who will accrue prestige from the increased ceremonial visits this road will facilitate, as well as the prestige of 'claiming' the land by guiding the location of the road across it.

It has already been noted that the Christians in several Western Desert communities prevented the 'churches' (which are really large halls) from being used by young people for recreational purposes. In other instances, adult desires have priority. In several Western Desert communities, for example, where the proportion of the population under the age of nineteen varies between 41 and 55 per cent, the allocation of funding and resources is invariably directed away from this age group. Many of these communities have no basketball courts and poor quality ovals, no recreation halls or sports equipment such as weights, no drop-in centres with pool tables or music. Despite this, major developments are taking place involving resource allocation: fully equipped roadhouses to capture the tourist traffic have been built near Giles and Warburton; a large new store complex has been built at Wingellina; and a police holding cell and courthouse has been built at Warburton.

Several communities have equipment or facilities which are, for various reasons, underutilised. Warakurna near Giles has a trampoline which is kept locked away because of lack of staff to supervise its use, and Blackstone has a small swimming pool which sometimes remains unfilled, also because of the absence of supervisory staff. Three communities in the region own buildings earmarked by local church groups which have prohibited their use for recreation or entertainment purposes. However, Warburton now has a large open-air swimming pool, built partly out of community funds. At Blackstone a recreation hall with a cement floor is used for roller skating by young people and 'in-house' movies are also shown there.

In communities which have no basketball, no recreation hall, poor ovals, no BMX bike tracks, no swimming pools, no television, no musical instruments and no rock groups, adults still successfully obtain funding to buy vehicles, for Bible Camps, outstations, traditional dance performances, festivals, arts and crafts and sometimes even overseas trips. While individual adults often spend freely on material items for their young kin (cassette players, BMX bikes), when it comes to the allocation of larger amounts of community funds, young people are rarely catered for. This is not surprising in view of their powerless position — they have no committees or councils to lobby for their needs, and no way of representing their interests. Because of this young people are never mobilised to act together except when they join sporting teams, or school-directed activities — and sniffing groups. Young people are also subordinate in social status — they cannot begin to accrue religious knowledge and the associated prestige until they are inducted into adulthood. For some, this process does not begin until a youth is eighteen or twenty years of age. It is hardly surprising, then, that they seek prestige elsewhere, either through their devotion to petrol sniffing or gang membership, or through moving around from settlement to settlement. Their power is exerted through starting affrays and by the provocation of fear.

There are other areas of social inaction within communities. For example, little attention is paid to the 'cultural' resources available to people. There are several so-called traditional forms of social control which are not commonly used to deal with sniffing, such as shaming. At present shaming appears to work against community welfare and in favour of the adolescents who use petrol. In parts of Arnhem Land there exists a powerful mechanism which is widely used on other occasions in order to inhibit certain activities. This is the use of 'cursing' — the placing of a prohibitive taboo on a person or an activity. The excessive use of cursing can be problematic as it has the power to reduce many community activities and facilities to a standstill. Ngukurr even passed resolutions (in the context of the Australian Law Reform Commission's inquiries into Aboriginal customary laws) stating that the 'placing of a Sacred Taboo' was a wrong thing to do and that those who placed such taboos should be made to pay compensation (Law Reform Commission 1986, 329). Nevertheless, in other communities this sanction is widely used — but never for the wrongful use of petrol or to assist an individual who wishes to abstain from petrol use. Aboriginal people in many regions feel that their powers to implement the punitive aspects of their own Law have been curtailed, as indeed they have. One Council chairman in Arnhem Land explained (personal communication):

> The elders are not real strict any more. A long time ago they was real strict. But you got two laws now: white law and Aboriginal law. If you punish someone 'seriously' then you go to court. If that law can be given back to control young people, through ceremony way, without white law interfering... . Before, elders told boys not to steal, do what we tell you, old men are going to watch you, you can't say bad words to your sister or brother. If elders spear or growl you, you can't talk back. We might spear you on the spot, or take you away.

There are, even so, other 'ceremonial' avenues within which controlling sanctions could be activated. In some cases this is already occurring, for example, during ritual performances at an east Arnhem community in September 1987 (associated with a deceased person) the young boys were instructed to keep the rules, and were specifically warned not to sniff petrol. If they 'did bad things', I was told, they must pay compensation. Another person described the ceremony as being 'like a school, teaching kids not to do this or that'. Ceremonies such as this one involved people from Beswick, Numbulwar, Ngukurr, Urapunga, Castello, Groote Eylandt and Borroloola — that is, covering an interlocking group of communities, some with petrol-sniffing youth, and some without. There are four 'culturally appropriate' avenues open to Aborigines in this region then: shaming, cursing, ceremonial instruction, and the imposition of compensation payments. The use of traditional healing techniques with petrol sniffers seems to be rare in Australia, although in one case an Aboriginal sniffer from a western New South Wales town was treated by an Aboriginal practitioner using smoke and the massage of the boy's feet (J Eggmolesse, personal communication). This is in stark contrast to the innovative use of native healing practices which is taking place in North America.

OVERSEAS INTERVENTIONS

Among native peoples in North America interventions into substance abuse have been devised that involve indigenous healing techniques. These include the use of sweat-lodge ceremonies, the peyote cult, drumming, herbalists, shamans and medicine men, and societies such as the Indian Shaker Church. The (United States) National Institute on Drug Abuse has published a booklet of tribal legends which can be used as prevention/education material. They tell stories of crises of adolescence and problem solving, none directly discussing drug use in itself (United States Department of Health, Education and Welfare 1978). The State Working Party on Petrol Sniffing has produced a booklet taking a similar approach, with illustrations telling stories of risk-taking and foolhardiness (State Working Party on Petrol Sniffing 1988).

While North American treatment programs for native drug and alcohol abusers are often based on non-native concepts such as Alcoholics Anonymous and psychological counselling, there is a growing realisation that many of these models alienate their native clients. In addition those with experience of inhalant abusers stress the particularly intransigent nature of this drug use and the length of time necessary for detoxification and recovery. Consequently, some programs using traditional medicine are being developed which direct their attention specifically to sniffers. For example, a group of Anishinabe (Ojibwa) healers associated with a district hospital in northwestern Ontario, Canada, have adapted and extended their existing native healers program to an innovative treatment system for sniffers. The program includes sniffers and their families and takes the form of a traditional medicine camp involving detoxification, purification (using the sweat-lodge), healing and unification ceremonies. The approach is based on the notion that the native sniffer needs to be exposed to a daring alternative as a means of counteracting the strong elements which support the practice of sniffing. Some of the traditional practices are intense and require endurance and determination. The program has the support of hospital physicians and local agencies.

Some native-controlled drug and alcohol treatment centres also emphasise native cultural values — what is termed 'traditionalism' — while allowing clients to follow other models (such as Alcoholics Anonymous or Christian spirituality) if they so choose. This neutral approach has been taken in some instances because of the ideological split between 'traditionalist' and church-based Indian groups in Canada. Nevertheless, there is an overall emphasis on Indian culture, language survival and the place of respected 'elders' in tackling the problem of substance abuse and in other helping agencies which are native-run.

Joan Weibel-Orlando (1989) has recently offered a critique of cultural relativism in substance abuse interventions and of many cross-cultural studies of addiction, suggesting that anthropologists may perpetuate myths which exaggerate the powers of local healers and underestimate the responsibility of governments. She reminds us that we still do not know if any sort of intervention, conventional or indigenous, works at all or for long periods of time. On a practical level, she proposes that social scientists are in a position to put forth the notion that total and lifelong abstinence is not always a culturally appropriate goal for intervention. She says (Weibel-Orlando 1989, 152):

> In fact, the abuse/intervention/recovery/use and abuse cycles which longitudinal research allows us to observe may be an indigenously developed self-regulatory pattern upon which institutional interventions can be modelled so as to afford them more cultural relevancy...perhaps one...goal can be the lengthening of the periods of abstinence, quiescence, and moderation.

On a pragmatic level, in a review of fifty Indian substance abuse programs, she analyses and summarises the most viable interventions, concluding that:

1. they were all self-generated, that is, a critical mass of the members of a certain community decided among themselves 'to do something';

2. they all had officiating or orienting charismatic role model initiators;

3. they all involved the recovering clients in ongoing therapy and interaction with the group both as healers and clients; and

4. they all saw themselves as a social entity.

Apart from emphasising the role of leaders, contemporary Canadian Indian literature on drug abuse interventions also emphasises 'the community' and its responsibility for dealing with these problems. This approach has arisen out of an attitude to social problems similar to that in many Australian Aboriginal communities (Draper 1985, 17):[3]

> They would always say: 'there's a child sniffing, Children's Aid should do something about it'. 'There's a boy, he's breaking windows — where's the police?' It was never what could be done in the community itself to stop it before it happened.

Community-based interventions taking place in Canada include youth groups in each community which meet two or three times a week and talk to each other on a tele-conference calling system each month. These tele-conference meetings keep group activities going and the youth offer support and assistance to each other. Youth conferences involving participants from each community are also held, which include workshops on suicide, alcohol and drugs. These workshops let the youth look at themselves and decide what they could and should do for each other. In a one-off experiment a youth caravan with a staff of workers travelled to communities for a stay of four days in each. In the communities, workshops were held on topics such as computers and videos, as well as cultural games, traditional games, drama, recreation and peer counselling. 'Once you leave the community, people realise that they have to do it on their own if they want to have things' (Northern Youth in Crisis 1985).

A notable feature of recent Canadian petrol-sniffing cases has been the sense of urgency which has prompted direct interventions known as the 'community intercept model' — an urgency arising out of chronic and widespread petrol sniffing among entire families and a high rate of suicide among young people. One writer describes the situation in a native community in Ontario and how residents dealt with it (Draper 1985, 18–19):

> Of the children under 16, approximately 60 were in care in Children's Aid Society, 58 were under the supervision of probation services, and one half of those were in training schools. Of the young adults, at least 25 were under supervision by probation and parole services. Of 77 total families, 25 had problems with alcohol and glue sniffing. At least 65 youths were involved in glue sniffing on a regular basis. Fifty percent of the population had alcohol problems. Over the previous two-year period, there had been 15 violent deaths. Over the previous five-year period, 80 per cent of all deaths on the reserve were violent — only 20 per cent were natural — a rather staggering and terrifying situation. ...There was peer pressure to sniff. Almost

every kid sniffed. Sniffing became the thing because gas [gasoline, petrol] is cheaper than alcohol.

Some community members decided to start a patrol, and every time they saw someone with petrol, or someone drunk, the patrols intervened, sending the individual home or making sure they were not in physical danger. Draper (1985, 19) says bluntly,

> Intrusion into people's lives. That is what intervention is. You are stepping into their private life. It was quite a serious change in many ways. However, the people knew that the state of the community was so bad that if something didn't happen, many youngsters and elders would die.

Draper (1985, 19) goes on to describe how concerned residents set up a crisis team:

> Many of them had records, but that was not the critical thing. The critical thing was interest in the community and a desire to improve it. The band council passed a resolution that the program and its members had the right to intervene in critical situations. They had the right, for example, to take a youth to the crisis centre. The duties of the crisis team members included patrolling the community, identifying crisis situations, conferring with community agencies, supervising emergency cases, diagnosing home situations, and referring cases to the appropriate agencies for follow-up.

THE INFLUENCE OF THE CATTLE INDUSTRY

While analysing the social epidemiology of petrol sniffing in Australia, I realised that there is one remarkable anomaly in the regional distribution of sniffing across South Australia, Western Australia and the Northern Territory. That anomaly suggests that the regions where petrol sniffing is not a serious problem, or where it rarely occurs at all, extend from northeast of Alice Springs across the Barkly Tablelands to the Arnhem Land border, west of Tennant Creek through the Victoria River district and across into the Kimberley and Pilbara regions of Western Australia. The issue that links all these areas, which contain a variety of Aboriginal populations of different sizes, is the cattle industry. Out of thirty-four major population centres in South Australia, Western Australia and the Northern Territory (excluding outstations) that reported petrol sniffing in 1985, only two (Neutral Junction and Ngukurr) are comprised of people who lived on cattle stations and worked in the cattle industry, or for whom the industry was a major component of their lives.

The substantial Aboriginal populations in these regions that do not have resident sniffers (ie without ruling out the occasional visiting sniffer) include Willowra, Utopia, Ali Curung, Lake Nash, Tennant Creek, Brunette Downs, Rockhampton Downs, Borroloola, Lajamanu, Daguragu, Victoria River Downs, Timber Creek, Amanbidji, Kununurra, Turkey Creek, Halls Creek, Derby, Strelley, Yandeearra, Port Hedland, and Roebourne. There are exceptions, where there has been some cattle enterprise on the land which has marginally involved Aborigines, and where petrol sniffing is or has been prevalent. Oenpelli, for example, had a government-run cattle station, but was also a CMS Mission (McGrath 1987, 109). Yuendumu has a cattle company, which in 1978 employed eleven stockworkers (Young 1981, 83). Haasts Bluff has a small enterprise. There was some pastoral development in the far north of South Australia on the fringes of what are now the Pitjantjatjara Lands, but Aboriginal people were not intimately involved, and the area proved so dry as to make success in the cattle industry impossible (Hope 1983, 154). Ngukurr Aborigines worked droving cattle between 1945 and the late 1960s and the community straddles the borders of the 'old' cattle industry and Arnhem Land, established as a reserve in 1937.

The pastoral industry was a major employer of Aboriginal people from the turn of the century until the late 1960s, when Aboriginal stock workers were brought under the provisions of the Cattle Station Industry Award.[4] As they had formed a cheap labour force up until that time, and were paid wages which were significantly below the award wage for white workers (and earlier had often received no wages at all), Aboriginal workers were laid off and effectively dispossessed of land on which their families had lived for generations.[5] Many were living on European leaseholds on their own land, and had successfully maintained contact with their land by working for stations located on it. In the 1930s, 80 per cent of all Aboriginal workers were to be found in the cattle industry, and on Northern Territory cattle stations 40 per cent of Aboriginal residents were employed — approximating the level of employment in the broader community in 1968 (Stevens 1974, 56). While Frank Stevens (1974) and Ronald and Catherine Berndt (1987) among others, have documented the harshness and cruelty to which Aboriginal workers were subjected, the unequal and discriminatory regimes of which they were victims and the injuries they sustained as a result of accidents, shootings and beatings, there is another side to the story which is now being told by Aborigines themselves with the help of oral historians (Sullivan 1983; Marshall 1988; McGrath 1987; Baker 1989).

In order to explore the proposition that there is a relationship between Aborigines influenced by the history of their association with the cattle industry and the absence of the practice of sniffing, we need to explore several key elements which characterise the impact of the cattle industry.

From the 1930s and before, in Arnhem Land and in Central Australia encompassing the far northwest of South Australia, Aboriginal people were increasingly under the influence of the settlements (government and mission-run). Northeast and northwest of Alice Springs and in the Victoria River Downs and the Kimberley, however, Aborigines were enmeshed in relationships of varying quality with European cattle enterprises. The stations were in fact dependent on Aboriginal labour, because the turnover of white staff was high, Europeans were often ignorant of the geography of the region, and Aboriginal labour was cheap and Aborigines worked hard. Stevens, interviewing European station managers in 1968, discovered that white stockmen often got lost and lacked courage, and that Aborigines were highly skilled, especially when dealing with wild cattle (1974, 139). Aborigines on cattle stations believed themselves to be superior to both mission and government reserve people, considering them to be poorly dressed, ill-housed and generally 'poor and dry' (McGrath 1987; Stevens 1974, 116). On the whole, Aborigines on cattle stations were better nourished than those in settlements and missions because they had access to fresh and plentiful meat and more cereals (Stevens 1974, 86). Weighing up conflicting opinions on the impact of the industry, Baker (1989) collected oral histories from Yanyuwa people in and around Borroloola in the Northern Territory. He proposed three main reasons why the cattle life was perceived positively by the Yanyuwa: association with the industry ensured the continuity of ceremonial life; it ensured the continuation of access to bush foods; and the industry valued Aboriginal skills.

Working on stations and particularly undertaking droving trips allowed Aboriginal men and women considerable autonomy and freedom of movement. Few activities could be supervised, so Aboriginal workers took responsibility for a wide range of jobs. Stockwork allowed people to visit and check up on their religious sites, maintaining links with their own land and visiting others, often carrying messages concerning ceremonial gatherings (Marshall 1988, 101, 191; McGrath 1987, 33, 39). Although local languages were spoken in stock camps, Kriol formed a lingua franca linking Kimberley Aborigines with the Roper region and beyond (McGrath 1987, 165). So-called 'traditional' culture was, in most cases, maintained. As McGrath points out, significant anthropological studies of station Aborigines by Stanner, Kaberry and Elkin were used to depict 'traditional' culture (1987, 168). The work involved a 'challenging variety of jobs' (Stevens 1974, 120): mustering; branding; bore, pump and windmill work; fencing; and shifting and droving cattle. Women were stock riders, drovers and fence builders too, often carrying their children strapped around their bodies. Yanyuwa men told Baker they liked the work because 'You knew what you were doing'; today the work available at Borroloola is menial — picking up rubbish (Baker 1989).

So how does all this relate to social circumstances in the 1970s and 1980s — social circumstances that appear to offer some protection, as it were, from the chronic use of petrol? There are five factors which could be influential: the internalisation of European values by Aborigines; the development of Aboriginal adult self-esteem; the small size of cattle communities; a secure male identity; and the perpetuation of identification with a cattle industry ethos.

Both Aboriginal men and women were literally 'broken in' by pastoralists (McGrath 1987, 62), with hidings and threats of punishment to make them work properly. The girls were often 'reared up' (as they say) by the European station women, who taught them to speak English, to wash and keep their clothes clean, to lay tables, iron, embroider and knit. The internalisation of European values was, to some extent, forced upon those working for station managers. 'Our old mother', recalled one, 'used to teach us, bashing us all the time…if we kids loafed around she would get into us or call the boss' (McGrath 1987, 116). John Watson told Marshall (1988, 232),

> We all had our jobs to do and if we didn't do them we got a hiding. But they [parents] always explained the reason why we got a hiding. We were disciplined in a good way, we knew who our bosses were. We learned from both sides, the Aboriginal and the Kartiya [white]… . I know that in the bigger communities the kids are getting outside the control of their parents.… My parents were very strong. If I started answering back I got a clip over the ear! That's the sort of discipline I'd like to see brought back.

As Baker points out, among the Borroloola people corporal punishment had been to some extent part of pre-European life — disputes were settled by fights — and there was some respect for 'hard' bosses as long as they were fair (Baker 1989). Older men complain that things are too easy nowadays. Chainsaws, for example, 'make people lazy…they're bringing in a really easy way now' (Marshall 1988, 54; see Rowse 1987, 90). While these statements echo the perennial 'It's not like it was in our day' theme, they still communicate the extent to which stockworkers came to accept the European notion that children (and Aborigines — who were 'childlike') needed to be brought under the control of adults (and Europeans) by physical coercion if necessary. Of course 'inside' Aborigines, those who had already been 'tamed', came to accept pastoralists' views that the 'outsiders' were wild and uncontrollable (see Rowse 1987); some assisted in tracking down the 'wild' ones. There are indications from these scattered accounts that Aborigines working on white-managed stations came to reflect some of the attitudes and actions of whites and in turn communicated these to their children — slackness and 'answering back' were not tolerated, judging by these accounts.

McGrath writes that 'Strictness and a high expectation of stockmen were part of being a "proper cattleman" to the Aboriginal way of thinking' (1987, 37). There was often equality of work between black and white, even if a yawning social chasm existed after hours (Stevens 1974, 20). The skills of Aborigines were of value to Europeans and workers constantly learned a range of new skills. Aborigines at Amanbidji (east of Kununurra) told me in 1987 that Reg Durack, for whom they worked, could never have succeeded in his cattle station if it had not been for them. This realisation means that there was, and is, a sense of self-esteem among Aboriginal pastoral workers.

During the 1930s, 1940s and 1950s, when Aboriginal populations in other areas were becoming centralised (either voluntarily or involuntarily) by missions and settlements into groups of 200 people or more, cattle station communities were generally much smaller than this. Added to this was a low birth rate in some areas (as a result of disease and malnutrition) and sometimes there were few young children. At Limbunya, McGrath notes, there were only three young children (1987, 137). Station managers left the 'blacks camp' alone on the whole, so that there was less interference in camp life and in disputes than there was in the settlements, where missionaries frequently intervened in fights and marriage arrangements. While under stress from other factors, people on cattle stations were not subjected to the tensions of living at close quarters with hundreds of others (see McKnight 1986). Presumably, when there was trouble, people were forced to deal with it themselves, for visits from patrol officers and government officials appear to have been infrequent.

Stevens remarks bluntly that among the young, childhood ended as early as nine years of age: 'By twelve or thirteen it was expected that the boys wanted to learn more about the cattle business...he was lifted into the saddle' (1974, 114). Only a small proportion of properties had schools — in Stevens's survey only thirty out of 210 stations had. Attitudes towards schooling were ambivalent by all accounts: 'They don't teach him much — just spellem name that's all' (Stevens 1974, 149; see Marshall 1988, 231). Male prestige was associated with bringing in meat — this is certainly the case among desert people, and Baker refers to this among Borroloola people as well (1989). Dugong, kangaroo or bullock, either wild meat or beef, was brought in throughout the cattle period — and working cattle in itself constituted an economic activity. Many other aspects of cattle work were deemed to be associated with manhood by Aboriginal people. McGrath (1987, 167) points out that

Ability with cattle was a highly prized skill, and the potential initiate had to prove himself agile with horses to be accepted on equal terms.... . Handling animals was an essential skill for survival in the changed environment; in the new economy it was just as important as ability with a spear.

Some, though by no means all, Aboriginal people in the major pastoral regions have been able to maintain their association with cattle work through small government-funded projects involving mustering and fencing (eg at Ngukurr), and with Aboriginal Development Corporation and other funding have purchased or leased cattle stations of their own (eg Amanbidji, Yandeearra, Willowra). In these cases, older people recognise the urgency of establishing their own enterprises before skills are lost (McGrath 1987, 167). Describing one such enterprise Ivan Watson told Marshall (1988, 159) of a Kimberley project:

Once those horses were on the place those lads flocked back here, regardless of the fact that we couldn't pay them. We had all those horses broken in within six weeks.... . I want to see those young fellas that stick with us get something out of the station in due course. They're showing all the old fellas here that we can make a go of the place.

Modern economic exigencies now mean that helicopters are used for mustering and European bull-catchers are often hired together with their equipment. Droving has been replaced by transportation by road. Even on cattle stations where this occurs, there is still a core of young men who have learned how to ride and are being taught horse-breaking (eg at Amanbidji). Kim McKenzie, while film-making at Robinson River in the Gulf country, Northern Territory, reported that the ambition of young boys there was unequivocally 'to be a ringer' when they grew up (K McKenzie, personal communication).[6] Young and old men with cattle associations wear the style of clothing associated with pastoral work — 'flash' satin shirts, flamboyant Akubras and leather boots. At rodeos Aborigines from surrounding districts are much in evidence.

In none of this discussion is there a single, simple factor to explain why young men and young women brought up on the modern, attenuated version of the cattle stations, or on their periphery, have not become involved in social groupings associated with petrol sniffing. Nor is it clear why, or how, the experiences of the parents and grandparents of the present generation should combine in a way that has prevented the establishment of this drug use. Alcohol is used by these people, especially those living close to or on the fringes of towns such as Fitzroy Crossing, Halls Creek and Kununurra. The fact remains that for a variety of possible reasons, sniffing is not noted among these populations. What does the pastoral identity of these Aboriginal people represent? Perhaps first, and most importantly, people who were intimately involved with the cattle industry were engaged in productive activity. As Sibthorpe (1988, 336) notes, in a discussion of stress and ill-health among rural New South Wales Aborigines:

> The psychosocial meaning of unemployment to Aborigines remains to be investigated, as do the meaning of concepts of work and leisure. However, productive activity is the mainstay of daily life in all societies and there is no reason to suppose that it is any different for Aborigines.

The cattle industry was significant, not because it was 'work' (there are countless menial, repetitive and mundane opportunities for Aborigines to work) but because it was productive — an economic enterprise. It was, in a sense, a transformation of traditional economic activity — marshalling, capturing and killing edible meat animals. In the course of the actual labours associated with cattle, people were engaged in productive activities of other kinds: collecting bush food; tending sites and performing ceremonies (both associated with caring for the land and making it productive); and increasing and extending their range of ritual knowledge through contact with other language groups. These factors contribute to a sense of pride and self-esteem which has not been lost to the present generation. Second, the older people from strong cattle industry backgrounds today still have a sense of identity with the cattle ethic, and so do the young men and women who were too young to have participated fully in it themselves. They have, perhaps, been brought up in a 'tougher' environment where there has been less tolerance of adolescent cheek. Whatever liberal-minded Europeans may think, Aboriginal people on the whole consider that in an ideal world adults are superordinate to young people. In many regions, the fact of petrol sniffing and the power that it allows young people to have (because of intoxication, uncontrolled behaviour and the fearfulness of others) is now articulated in terms of the young having got 'on top' of the old. In Ngaanyatjarra regions, people frequently used a particular term for the petrol sniffers, *tunguntungunpa*, which means rebellious, disobedient or stubborn, according to one linguist (Hansen and Hansen 1977). Another translates it as unyielding, resistant or contrary (Goddard 1987). Wilf Douglas (another linguist) suggests arrogant and insolent as well (Douglas 1988). Local people when questioned replied they meant that the petrol sniffers were 'smart', they 'take over, themselves'. One man said they were 'In opposition — you know, like Mr Howard'.[7] These explanations make it clear that the adults consider these young people to be getting beyond themselves (posing a threat to the adults). Being 'smart' in this sense, is not a desired attribute. Those with experience of or access to cattle work have a chance to test out their smartness on wild bulls, by throwing steers, and by breaking in horses. Even though access to such work is now more restricted, we can hypothesise that, in some intangible way, in these populations self-esteem and male identity have remained intact, so that young people have not yet sought to express their personal autonomy through the act of petrol sniffing.

NOTES

1. The response to the use of kava — which is not in itself toxic — by a small proportion of Aboriginal people in one region, stands in stark contrast. Within a few years of its introduction to Arnhem Land in 1982, its use had been surveyed (Watson et al 1988), its physiological effects measured by nutritionists and physicians (Mathews et al 1988) and warning 'casualty reduction' pamphlets were distributed by the Northern Territory Health Department.

2. The State Working Party on Petrol Sniffing adopted this consciousness-raising approach in Western Australia in the late 1980s.

3. Children's Aid in Canada refers to the government child protection and welfare agency. In some instances native-run child and family services are now mandated by the federal government to undertake the role of the Children's Aid Society.

4. Equal wages were granted on 1 December 1968 (Stevens 1974, 205).

5. For example, Coniston Station used to employ thirty Aboriginal men, but in 1973 employed less than half that number at any one time (Stanley 1974).

6. A ringer is a stockman.

7. John Howard was then the leader of the federal Opposition.

CONCLUSION

This book began with the assertion that the different explanations mooted for the causes of substance abuse among Aborigines on the one hand, and non-Aborigines on the other, present some problems. There is a preoccupation with the search for causes because it is thought that if we 'really' knew why (in this case) young Aboriginal people sniff petrol, we could do something about it. There is, then, an unspoken assumption that it will be possible to solve this particular drug use problem, to eradicate it. It is probably more realistic to accept that there is a complex of factors at work; that for this reason we will be unable to state clearly the supposed reasons for sniffing; and that complete eradication of this drug use (and many others) is unlikely to occur. Young Aborigines form a large proportion of the present populations. Within ten years or so, these young people will have children of their own; some already have children, and drug use (of one form or another) will undoubtedly continue to be an issue. It has been established that the substance itself, petrol, is toxic. While occasional limited use causes few long-term ill-effects, prolonged and systematic inhalation of petrol vapours can produce symptoms requiring hospitalisation. It has been directly associated with at least thirty-five documented Aboriginal deaths over an eight-year period — more deaths than are caused by any other single volatile substance. The cost, in terms of long-term intellectual and motor impairment, is still unknown.

The findings of this study have ramifications both for the medical interventions currently being implemented with users, and for the popular understandings of the practice itself. In terms of the clinical symptomatology of petrol sniffing, I have raised the question of a possible overemphasis on the toxicity of lead in petrol with a concomitant underemphasis on the other toxic hydrocarbons contained in fuel. The symptoms associated with each are hard to distinguish, and hospital treatments in Australia are uncoordinated, so that physicians in one region take one approach, others elsewhere take another. I have avoided popular explanations which seek to find 'causes' for the practice, and instead have suggested that, in sniffing, young people are summoning up one of the few avenues of power available to them — the power to have autonomy over one's own body. Within this context, some who sniff exert control over themselves and others by using petrol as a means of losing weight and becoming thin. Others have found an identity of sorts by carefully stage-managing their dress, behaviour and musical tastes and identifying with gangs. By so doing they outrage both the concerned white staff of their communities and the norms of their own society. They resist, for as long as possible, being incorporated into the status quo offered them.

This study has also drawn attention to a previously unexplored question: why the young in some communities sniff petrol, while in others they do not? The most compelling explanation for the distribution of the practice is the historical and social context of the cattle industry. The regions where the cattle industry was, or still is, part of Aboriginal life have a low or non-existent incidence of petrol sniffing. Sniffing has taken root in some of the most 'tradition-oriented' of communities, on land owned under Australian law by Aboriginal people, and among people whose historic contact with whites has been through settlements administered by missionaries and government welfare agents. It has generally not become established in the populations who were associated with the pastoral industry, which was tolerant of mobility, economically sound and tested the skills of its Aboriginal workers.

The only feasible solutions lie in providing the set (the users) with a setting within which the drug is used either in a controlled and limited manner, or within which the opportunity and desire to use the drug are minimised. However, ritualised controls among drug users, which are often part of the setting for drug use, have not yet developed for this substance. As some of the evidence presented here shows, while individuals usually ultimately abandon the use of petrol, the practice has itself intensified over the years so that its current usage among chronic sniffers is qualitatively and quantitatively different from the use noted in the 1960s and early 1970s. The reasons for this absence of in-group controls are relatively simple. For many users there are still compelling reasons why they should engage in the practice in an habitual and committed way. It provides them with an opportunity to state their personal autonomy within an environment which otherwise provides them few such opportunities. It provides them with the opportunity to exploit the loopholes in the social system, while provoking complex feelings of guilt, shame and concern on the part of others bonded to them in the interpersonal realm. It provides them with power over others in a situation in which they are otherwise powerless, and in which adult priorities and desires are, at least partially, fulfilled. The drug use also allows users to express their resistance to incorporation in their own society, and to seek deliberately oppositional styles and behaviours designed to provoke response. It also enables them to reject white Australian values and concerns, and it offers an alternative reality to one which may be otherwise painful, despairing and empty.

As a result of curtailed social sanctions and disruption to social structures, the avenues whereby Aboriginal people may have been able to exert control have become constricted. These disruptions have not been responsible for the genesis of the use of petrol as a drug, but are probably associated with the entrenchment and proliferation of the practice. While most young people in our society probably experience similar crises and use drugs to solve similar problems, in the wider society they usually have at their disposal a broad range of material resources with which to create lifestyles to compete with the attractions of drug use. They also have access to more treatment facilities. However, while treatment and counselling may be appropriate in some cases for users of petrol, not only are such facilities sorely lacking at present in the regions associated with petrol use, they are not the complete solution. Petrol sniffing, like heroin use, is maintained in the immediate neighbourhood of users, and that is where it must be combated. Pearson (1987) nominates decent housing and jobs as some of the elements found wanting in the area he studied; in the Aboriginal context perhaps the vital element is meaningful productive activity, not necessarily paid 'work'. All human societies need meaningful productive activity and there is no evidence to suggest that Aboriginal society is any different. There must be compelling and competing activities available to combat petrol sniffing, for people abandon a dysfunctional drug use only when it begins to interfere with too many other valued aspects of their lives. If there are no other valued aspects to life, then there is simply no compulsion to abstain.

In an assessment of the elements that inhibit the control of petrol sniffing, we can identify several different levels of inaction. On a national level, despite the creation of policy statements about the practice and the conduct of a Senate Select Committee of inquiry, there is still no one individual or department responsible for petrol-sniffing programs, for monitoring successes and failures, or for collating data on interventions, prevalence, morbidity and mortality. There is no-one whose responsibility it is to work on the production of locally made videos and educational material; no-one who can discover an approach emanating from one region and suggest that its principles could be applied elsewhere. Despite several attempts, the state and federal government departments have still not fully coordinated a consistent approach to petrol sniffing. Indeed, action on this particular drug use could be said to have fallen victim to federal–state and inter-departmental rivalries.

The Aboriginal communities themselves still suffer from the excessive complexity of the government agencies with whom they must deal during any applications for funding. Budgeting is done in advance; they have no access to emergency funds which could disburse small amounts for local projects, and therefore provide a fast-moving response to a community initiative arising from local motivation to act. Competition for resources is high, a situation which tends to lead people away from mutual cooperation and towards individual concerns. The communities' motivation to act decisively in the context of petrol sniffing, while heavily influenced by historical and cultural factors, is also impeded by political and economic structures. As documented, adult priorities have precedence in community affairs, and the young are rarely considered. Young people have no voice in the communities, and while cherished and held in high regard by Aboriginal people, are relatively powerless to influence community or Council decisions, let alone those of governments.

The research documented here has made it clear that petrol sniffing is not uniformly practised among remote and rural settlement dwellers, and that the entrenched use of this volatile substance as a drug is restricted to some specific regions of Australia. Why this should be so is a matter of conjecture, but it has at least been possible to suggest that a quality in the lifestyle, or in the life events, of Aboriginal people who have historically been part of the cattle industry has assisted those people to prevent the development of sniffing among their children. In view of the common assumptions about the genesis of drug and alcohol abuse among Aboriginal peoples (both in Australia and overseas), it is ironic that it is the Aboriginal populations associated with the cattle industry which have resisted petrol sniffing; even in the 1990s, these groups rarely have secure title to their land as many ex-mission and welfare settlement populations do. The history of the dispossession and harsh treatment of cattle station people has been widely documented. Still, the setting in these cases has served to provide environments within which this drug use is not favoured. The setting has interacted with the individual desires and expectations of young adults to help them avoid becoming interested in the strange sensations offered by sniffing. Because the practice has failed to develop among a 'critical' group of a particular size and influence in these areas, there is, as a consequence, no consistent pressure for adolescents to engage in it, or to transform an occasional experiment into an continuing activity.

REFERENCES

Ahern, K.B.
    1987   South Australian Coroner's Report, 23 April, South Australian Coroner's Office.

Akerman, K. and P. Bindon
    1986   Love Magic and Style Changes Within One Class of Love Magic Objects, *Oceania* 57(1), 22–32.

Albrecht, P.G.E.
    1974   The Social and Psychological Reasons for the Alcohol Problem Among Aborigines. In B.S. Hetzel, M. Dobbin, L. Lippmann and E. Eggleston (eds), *Better Health for Aborigines?*, University of Queensland Press, St Lucia.

Alexander, K., C. Watson and J. Fleming
    1987   *Kava in the North*, North Australia Research Unit, Darwin.

Alice Springs Hospital
    1986   *Protocol for the Treatment of Petrol Sniffers*, mimeograph, Alice Springs Hospital, Alice Springs.

Alroe, M.
    1988   A Pygmalion Complex among Missionaries: The Catholic Case in the Kimberley. In T. Swain and D.B. Rose (eds), *Aboriginal Australians and Christian Missions*, the Australian Association for the Study of Religions at the South Australian College of Advanced Education, Sturt Campus, South Australia.

Altman, J.C.
    1982   Hunter-gatherers and the State: The Economic Anthropology of the Gunwinggu of North Australia, PhD thesis, Australian National University, Canberra.

    1987   *Hunter-gatherers Today: An Aboriginal Economy in North Australia*, Australian Institute of Aboriginal Studies, Canberra.

Bain, M.
    1974   Alcohol Use and Traditional Social Controls in Aboriginal Society. In B.S. Hetzel, M. Dobbin, L. Lippmann and E. Eggleston (eds), *Better Health for Aborigines?*, University of Queensland Press, St Lucia.

Baker, R.
    1989   Land Is Life: Continuity Through Change for the Yanyuwa of the Northern Territory of Australia, PhD thesis, University of Adelaide, Adelaide.

Barber, J.G., J. Punt and J. Albers
    1988   Alcohol and Power on Palm Island, *Australian Journal of Social Issues* 23(2), 87–101.

Barnes, G.
1980   *Northern Sniff: The Epidemiology of Drug Use among Indian, White and Metis Adolescents*, Department of Psychiatry and Psychology, University of Manitoba, Winnipeg.
1985   Gasoline Sniffing, *Revue Canadienne d'Economie Familiale* 35(3), 144–58.

Bass, M.
1970   Sudden Sniffing Death, *Journal of the American Medical Association* 212(12), 2075–79.

Bastian, P.
1979   Coronary Heart Disease in Tribal Aborigines: The West Kimberley Survey, *Australia and New Zealand Journal of Medicine* 9(3), 284–92.

Beauvais, F. and S. LaBoeff
1985   Drug and Alcohol Abuse: Intervention in American Indian Communities, *International Journal of the Addictions* 20(1), 139–71.

Beckett, J.
1964   Aborigines, Alcohol, and Assimilation. In M. Reay (ed), *Aborigines Now: New Perspective in the Study of Aboriginal Communities*, Angus and Robertson, Sydney.

Bern, J.
1979   Politics in the Conduct of a Secret Male Ceremony, *Journal of Anthropological Research* 35(1), 47–60.

Berndt, R.M
1976   Territoriality and the Problem of Demarcating Sociocultural Space. In N. Peterson (ed), *Tribes and Boundaries in Australia*, Australian Institute of Aboriginal Studies, Canberra.

Berndt, R.M. and C.H. Berndt
1987   *End of an Era: Aboriginal Labour in the Northern Territory*, Australian Institute of Aboriginal Studies, Canberra.

Biles, D.
1983   *A Research Report: Groote Eylandt Prisoners*, Australian Institute of Criminology, Canberra.

Black, P.
1967   Mental Illness due to the Voluntary Inhalation of Petrol Vapour, *Medical Journal of Australia* 8 July, 70–71.

Boeckx, R.L., B. Postl and F.J. Coodin
1977   Gasoline Sniffing and Tetraethyl Lead Poisoning in Children, *Pediatrics* 60(2), 140–45.

Bonnheim, M. and M. Korman
1985   Family Interaction and Acculturation in Mexican–American Inhalant Users, *Journal of Psychoactive Drugs* 17(1), 25–33.

Bourdieu, P.
1977 *Outline of a Theory of Practice*, Cambridge University Press, Cambridge.

Bos, R.
1988 The Dreaming and Social Change in Arnhem Land. In T. Swain and D.B. Rose (eds), *Aboriginal Australians and Christian Missions*, the Australian Association for the Study of Religions at the South Australian College of Advanced Education, Sturt Campus, South Australia.

Brady, M.
1985a *Children without Ears: Petrol Sniffing in Australia*, Drug and Alcohol Services Council, Adelaide.

1985b Aboriginal Youth and the Juvenile Justice System. In A. Borowski and J.M. Murray (eds), *Juvenile Delinquency in Australia*, Methuen, North Ryde.

1987 Dealing with Disorder: Strategies of Accommodation among the Southern Pitjantjatjara, Australia, MA thesis, Australian National University, Canberra.

1989 Number One for Action, *Australian Aboriginal Studies* 1, 62–63.

Brady, M. and R. Morice
1982 Aboriginal Adolescent Offending Behaviour: Report to the Criminology Research Council by Western Desert Project, Flinders University of South Australia, Adelaide (also held in the Australian Institute of Criminology Library, Canberra).

Brady, M. and K. Palmer
1984 *Alcohol in the Outback*, North Australia Research Unit, Darwin.

Brady, M. and K. Palmer
1988 Dependency and Assertiveness: Three Waves of Christianity among Pitjantjatjara People at Ooldea and Yalata. In T. Swain and D.B. Rose (eds), *Aboriginal Australians and Christian Missions*, the Australian Association for the Study of Religions at the South Australian College of Advanced Education, Sturt Campus, South Australia.

Brody, H.
1975 *The People's Land: Eskimos and Whites in the Eastern Arctic*, Penguin, Harmondsworth, UK.

Brown, A.
1983 Petrol Sniffing Lead Encephalopathy, *New Zealand Medical Journal* 96(733), 421–22.

Brown, V.A., D. Manderson, M. O'Callaghan and R. Thomson
1986 *Our Daily Fix: Drugs in Australia*, Australian National University Press, Canberra.

Burbank, V.K.
　1980　　Some of the History, Custom and Law of the People of Numbulwar, manuscript, Australian Institute of Aboriginal and Torres Strait Islander Studies (AIATSIS) Library, Canberra.

　1988　　*Aboriginal Adolescence: Maidenhood in an Aboriginal Community*, Rutgers University Press, New Brunswick.

Burd, L., T.E. Shea and H. Knull
　1987　　'Montana Gin': Ingestion of Commercial Products Containing Denatured Alcohol among Native Americans, *Journal of Studies on Alcohol* 48(4), 388–89.

Carlini-Cotrim, B. and E.A. Carlini
　1988　　The Use of Solvents and Other Drugs among Children and Adolescents from a Low Socio-economic Background, *International Journal of Addictions* 23(11), 1145–56.

Carr, D.J. and S.G.M. Carr
　1981　　*People and Plants in Australia*, Academic Press, Sydney.

Carroll, E.
　1977　　Notes on the Epidemiology of Inhalants. In C.W. Sharp and M.L. Brehm (eds), *Review of Inhalants: Euphoria to Dysfunction*, NIDA Research Monograph 15, National Institute on Drug Abuse, Division of Research, Rockville, Maryland.

Carroll, H. and G. Abel
　1973　　Chronic Gasoline Inhalation, *Southern Medical Journal* 66(12), 1429–30.

Cawte, J.
　1988　　Macabre Effects of a 'Cult' for Kava, *Medical Journal of Australia* 148, 6 June, 545–46.

Cheek, D.B., G.H. McIntosh, V. O'Brien, D. Ness and R.C. Green
　1989　　Malnutrition in Aboriginal Children at Yalata, South Australia, *European Journal of Clinical Nutrition* 43, 161–68.

Chief Protector of Aborigines
　1911　　*Annual Report of the Chief Protector of Aborigines for Year 1910*, 59–1911, 22–23, Brisbane, Queensland.

Chisholm, J.J.
　1987　　Mobilization of Lead by Calcium Disodium Edetate, *American Journal of Diseases of Children* 141, December, 1256–57.

Church Missionary Society (CMS)
　various　CMS Monthly Reports, Roper River, Numbulwar, Angurugu, held at
　dates　　CMS field headquarters, Anglican Church of Australia, Diocese of the Northern Territory, Bagot Rd, Nightcliff, Northern Territory.

Cohen, A.
　1966　　*Deviance and Control*, Prentice-Hall, Englewood Cliffs, New Jersey.

Cole, K.
1980   *Dick Harris: Missionary to the Aborigines*, Keith Cole Publications, Victoria.

1984   *Fred Gray of Umbakumba*, Keith Cole Publications, Victoria.

Cole, M., D.N. Herndon, M.H. Desai and S. Abston
1986   Gasoline Explosions, Gasoline Sniffing: An Epidemic in Young Adolescents, *Journal of Burn Care and Rehabilitation* 7(6), 532–34.

Collmann, J.
1988   *Fringe-Dwellers and Welfare: The Aboriginal Response to Bureaucracy*, University of Queensland Press, St Lucia.

Commonwealth of Australia
1985   *Volatile Substance Abuse in Australia*, Senate Select Committee on Volatile Substance Fumes, Australian Government Publishing Service, Canberra.

1987   *Return to Country: The Aboriginal Homelands Movement in Australia*, House of Representatives Standing Committee on Aboriginal Affairs, Australian Government Publishing Service, Canberra.

1988   *Alcohol in Australia: A Summary of Related Statistics*, Department of Community Services and Health, Australian Government Publishing Service, Canberra.

1991   *Royal Commission into Aboriginal Deaths in Custody National Report*, Australian Government Publishing Service, Canberra.

Commonwealth Department of Community Services and Health
1988   *Statistics on Drug Abuse in Australia 1988*, Australian Government Publishing Service, Canberra.

Commonwealth Department of Health
1985   *Abuse of Volatile Substances, Information Paper 5: Petrol Inhalation*, Commonwealth Department of Health, Canberra.

Coombs, H.C., M.M. Brandl and W. Snowdon
1983   *A Certain Heritage*, Centre for Resource and Environmental Studies, Australian National University, Canberra.

Coulehan, J., W. Hirsch, J. Brillman, J. Sanandria, T.K. Welty, P. Colaiaco, A. Koros and A. Lober
1983   Gasoline Sniffing and Lead Toxicity in Navajo Adolescents, *Pediatrics* 71(1), 113–17.

Council for Aboriginal Alcohol Program Services (CAAPS)
nd   *Co-dependents Program*, mimeograph, Gordon Symonds Centre, Winnellie, Darwin.

Coutts, N.
1980   Petrol Sniffing: A Community Crisis, *Developing Education* 8(4), 4–6.

Cowlishaw, G.
 1982a   Family Planning, A Post-Contact Problem. In J. Reid (ed), *Body, Land and Spirit: Health and Healing in Aboriginal Society*, University of Queensland Press, St Lucia.
 1982b   Socialisation and Subordination among Australian Aborigines, *Man* 17 (new series), 492–507.

D'Abbs, P.
 1987   *Dry Areas, Alcohol and Aboriginal Communities: A Review of the Northern Territory Restricted Areas Legislation*, Department of Health and Community Services, Darwin.

Dalton-Morgan, D.
 1978   Petrol Sniffing. Papunya: A Community Solution, *Australian Crime Prevention Quarterly Journal* 1(1), 32–33.

Daniels, A. and R. Fazakerley
 1983   Solvent Abuse in the Central Pacific, *The Lancet* 1(8), 75.

De la Fuente, R.
 1983   Mexico: Inhalants and an Urban Terrain. In G. Edwards, A. Arif and J. Jaffe (eds), *Drug Use and Misuse: Cultural Perspectives*, Croom Helm, London and Canberra, and St. Martins Press, New York.

Department of Education, Employment and Training
 1989   Grants Worth $1m. to Help Save Aboriginal Languages, *Aboriginal News*, August.

Department of Health and Social Security
 1980   *Lead and Health: The Report of a DHSS Working Party on Lead in the Environment*, Her Majesty's Stationery Office, London.

Devanesen, D., M. Furber, D. Hampton, M. Honari, N. Kinmonth and H.G. Peach
 1986   *Health Indicators in the Northern Territory*, Department of Health, Darwin.

Dingle, A.E.
 1980   The Truly Magnificent Thirst: An Historical Survey of Australian Drinking Habits, *Historical Studies* 19(75), 227–49.

Douglas, W.H.
 1988   *An Introductory Dictionary of the Western Desert Language*, Institute of Applied Language Studies, Perth.

Draper, C.
 1985   *The Creation and Operation of Crisis Intervention Programs for Northern Youth: The Case of Grassy Narrows*, paper delivered to conference, Northern Youth in Crisis, Quebec, November 1985 Department of Continuing Studies, Simon Fraser University, British Columbia.

REFERENCES

Drew, L.R.H.
    1983   Drug-related Deaths in Australia from 1969 to 1980, *Australian Alcohol/Drug Review* 2(1), 47–53.

Eastwell, H.D.
    1979   Petrol Inhalation in Aboriginal Towns: Its Remedy, The Homelands Movement, *Medical Journal of Australia* 2, 8 September, 221–24.

Eckerman, A.K, B.H. Watts and P.A. Dixon
    1984   From Here to There: A Comparative Study of Aboriginal Rural–Urban Resettlement in Queensland and New South Wales, report to the Department of Aboriginal Affairs, Canberra.

Elkin, A.P.
    1931   The Social Organisation of South Australian Tribes, *Oceania* II(1), 44–73.

Elsegood, P.
    nd   *Petrol Sniffing: Is It a Problem*, mimeograph, Remote Area Team, Northern Territory Department of Community Welfare.

Empowering our People
    1990   'Lets talk about inhalant abuse', panel discussion, Fourth Annual National Native American Conference on Inhalant Abuse, October 29–31, Spokane, Washington.

Epstein, A.L.
    1984   The Experience of Shame in Melanesia: An Essay in the Anthropology of Affect, *Occasional Paper* 40, Royal Anthropological Institute of Britain and Ireland, London.

Erikson, K.T.
    1962   Notes on the Sociology of Deviance, *Social Problems* 9, 307–14.

Ferguson, D.
    1978   *Report on Petrol Sniffing at Amata, 11/9/78*, mimeograph, AIATSIS Library, Canberra.

Folds, R.
    1987   *Whitefella School*, Allen and Unwin, Sydney.

Fornazzari, L.
    1988   Clinical Recognition and Management of Solvent Abusers, *Internal Medicine for the Specialist* 9(6) June, 99–109.

Foucault, M.
    1979   *Discipline and Punish: The Birth of the Prison*, Vintage Books, New York.

Franks, C.
    1989   Preventing Petrol Sniffing in Aboriginal Communities, *Community Health Studies* XIII(1), 14–22.

Freeman, P.
　1985　Petrol Sniffing in Amata, South Australia. In Nganampa Health Council (ed), *Health Report*, Nganampa Health Council Inc, Alice Springs.

Gerritsen, R.
　1982　Outstations: Differing Interpretations and Policy Implications. In P. Loveday (ed), *Service Delivery to Outstations*, North Australia Research Unit, Darwin.

Gibson, M.
　1987　Anthropology and Tradition: A Contemporary Aboriginal Viewpoint, paper presented at Australian and New Zealand Association for the Advancement of Science (ANZAAS) conference, Peoples of the North, Townsville (also held in the AIATSIS Library).

Giese, H.C.
　1957　Tribal Analysis of Aboriginal School Children at the Following Schools: July/August 1957, undated letter and report to Prof. A.P. Elkin, Department of Aboriginal Affairs file 56/293(2), Northern Territory Welfare Branch, Northern Territory.

Gilroy, S.M.
　1976　Youthful Offenders at Groote Eylandt, *Legal Service Bulletin* December, 124–26.

Glass, B.
　1981　Lead Poisoning, *Patient Management* June, 41–50.

Goddard, C.
　1987　*A Basic Pitjantjatjara/Yankunytjatjara to English Dictionary*, Institute for Aboriginal Development, Alice Springs.

Gold, N.
　1963　Self-intoxication by Petrol Vapour Inhalation, *Medical Journal of Australia* October, 582–84.

Gracey, M.
　1977　Nutritional Problems of Australian Aborigines, *Proceedings of the Nutrition Society of Australia* 2, 11–16.

Grandjean, P.
　1983　Health Significance of Organolead Compounds. In M. Rutter and R. Russell Jones (eds), *Lead Versus Health*, John Wiley and Sons, London.
　1984　Organolead Exposures and Intoxications. In P. Grandjean (ed), *Biological Effects of Organolead Compounds*, CRC Press, USA.

Gray, A.
　1985　Limits for Demographic Parameters of Aboriginal Populations in the Past, *Australian Aboriginal Studies* 1985/no 1, 22–27.

Green, N.
　1983　*Desert School*, Fremantle Arts Centre Press, Fremantle.

Hall, D., J. Ramsey, M. Schwartz and D. Dookun
   1986   Neuropathy in a Petrol Sniffer, *Archives of Disease in Childhood* 61, 900–16.

Hall, R.
   1980   Aborigines, the Army and the Second World War in Northern Australia, *Aboriginal History* 4(1), 73–95.

Hamilton, A.
   1981   *Nature and Nurture: Aboriginal Child-Rearing in North-Central Arnhem Land*, Australian Institute of Aboriginal Studies, Canberra.

Hansen, K.C. and L.E. Hansen
   1977   *Pintupi and Luritja Dictionary*, Institute for Aboriginal Development, Alice Springs.

Harding, W.M. and N.E. Zinberg
   1977   The Effectiveness of the Subculture in Developing Rituals and Social Sanctions for Controlled Drug Use. In B.M. du Toit (ed), *Drugs, Rituals and Altered States of Consciousness*, A.A. Balkema, Rotterdam.

Harris, B.M.
   1988   *The Rise of Rascalism: Action and Reaction in the Evolution of Rascal Gangs*, Discussion Paper no 54, Institute of Applied Social and Economic Research, Boroko, Papua New Guinea.

Harris, S.
   1984   *Culture and Learning: Tradition and Education in North-east Arnhem Land*, Australian Institute of Aboriginal Studies, Canberra.

Harrison, L.
   1986   Diet and Nutrition in a Tiwi Community, PhD thesis, Australian National University, Canberra.

Hayward, L. and M. Kickett
   1988   An Analysis of Morbidity and Mortality in 1981–86 and the Prevalence of Petrol Sniffing in Aboriginal Children in the Western Desert Region in 1987, Health Department, Western Australia Drug Data Collection Unit, Perth.

Hayward-Ryan, T.
   1979   Petrol Sniffing amongst Juveniles in the Northern Territory: An Interim Review, Department of Community Development, Community Welfare Division, minute, through Director to Secretary, 26 February 1979, AIATSIS Library, Canberra.

Hebdige, D.
   1979   *Subculture: The Meaning of Style*, Methuen, London.

Hedges, J.B.
   1986   *Community Justice Systems and Alcohol Controls*, Aboriginal Affairs Planning Authority, Perth.

Hiatt, L.R.
  1965 *Kinship and Conflict: A Study of an Aboriginal Community in Northern Arnhem Land*, Australian National University Press, Canberra.

Higginbotham, H.N.
  1984 Culture Accommodation of Mental Health Services and Beyond. In H.N. Higginbotham (ed), *Third World Challenge to Psychiatry*, University of Hawaii Press, Honolulu.

Holden, N.L. and P.H. Robinson
  1988 Anorexia Nervosa and Bulimia Nervosa in British Blacks, *British Journal of Psychiatry* 152, 544–49.

Hollobon, J.
  1987 Return to Native Traditions Works, *The Journal* (Addiction Research Foundation, Toronto) 1, 8 December.

Hope, D.A.C.
  1983 Dreams Contested: A Political Account of Relations between South Australia's Pitjantjatjara and the Government, 1961–1981, PhD thesis, School of Social Sciences, Flinders University of South Australia, Adelaide.

Hughes, R.
  1987 *The Fatal Shore*, Pan, London.

Hunt, H.
  1981 Alcoholism among Aboriginal People, *Medical Journal of Australia* (special supp.) 1(2), 1–3.

Institute for Aboriginal Development
  1985 *Current Distribution of Central Australian Languages*, map, Institute for Aboriginal Development, Alice Springs.

Jaffe, J.
  1983 What Counts as a 'Drug Problem'? In G. Edwards, A. Arif and J. Jaffe (eds), *Drug Use and Misuse, Cultural Perspectives*, Croom Helm, London and Canberra, and St Martin's Press, New York.

Japanangka, D.L. and P. Nathan
  1983 *Settle Down Country*, Central Australian Aboriginal Congress, Alice Springs, and Kibble Books, Melbourne.

Kaelen, C., C. Harper and B. Vieira
  1986 Acute Encephalopathy and Death due to Petrol Sniffing: Neuropathological Findings, *Australian and New Zealand Journal of Medicine* 16(6), 804–7.

Kamien, M.
  1975 A Survey of Drug Use in a Part-Aboriginal Community, *Medical Journal of Australia* 1 March, 261–64.

Kaufman, A.
1973 Gasoline Sniffing among Children in a Pueblo Indian Village, *Pediatrics* 51(6), 1060–64.

Keeffe, K.
1989 Curriculum Development in Aboriginal Studies: A Yanangu Case Study, *Australian Aboriginal Studies* 1989/no 1, 36–44.

Keenlyside, R.A.
1984 The Gasoline-sniffing Syndrome. In P. Grandjean (ed), *Biological Effects of Organolead Compounds*, CRC Press, USA.

Kohn, M.
1987 *Narcomania: On Heroin*, Faber and Faber, London.

Kunitz, S.J. and J.E. Levy
1974 Changing Ideas of Alcohol Use among Navaho Indians, *Quarterly Journal of Studies on Alcohol* 35(1), 243–59.

Kunitz, S.J., J.E. Levy, C.L. Odoroff and J. Bollinger
1971 The Epidemiology of Alcoholic Cirrhosis in Two South-Western Indian Tribes, *Quarterly Journal of Studies on Alcohol* 32(3), 706–20.

Laurie, A. and A. McGrath
1985 I Was a Drover Once Myself: Amy Laurie of Kununurra. In I. White, D. Barwick and B. Meehan (eds), *Fighters and Singers*, George Allen and Unwin, Sydney.

Law Reform Commission
1986 *The Recognition of Aboriginal Customary Laws*, Law Reform Commission report no 31, Australian Government Publishing Service, Canberra.

Lee A.
1988 Apparent Dietary Intake in Remote Aboriginal Communities. In *Menzies School of Health Research Annual Report 1987–1988*, Menzies School of Health Research, Darwin.

Legislative Assembly of the Northern Territory
1991 *Measures for Reducing Alcohol Use and Abuse in the Northern Territory*, Interim Report of the Sessional Committee on Use and Abuse of Alcohol by the Community, Northern Territory Government Printer, Darwin.

Lepowsky, M.
1982 A Comparison of Alcohol and Betelnut Use on Vanatinai (Sudest Island). In M. Marshall (ed), *Through a Glass Darkly: Beer and Modernization in Papua New Guinea*, Monograph 18, Institute of Applied Social and Economic Research, Boroko, Papua New Guinea.

Levitt, D.
1981 *Plants and People: Aboriginal Uses of Plants on Groote Eylandt*, Australian Institute of Aboriginal Studies, Canberra.

Lindstrom, L. (ed)
    1987   *Drugs in Western Pacific Societies: Relations of Substance*, University Press of America, Lanham.

Lisansky-Gomberg, E.S.
    1989   On Terms Used and Abused: The Concept of 'Codependency', *Drugs and Society* 3 (3–4), 113–32.

Lowe, H.
    1988   Recovery of Traditional Aboriginal Family Systems: Adaption or Assimilation?, paper presented to International Congress, Alcohol, other Drugs and the Family, Sydney.

Lund, S., R. Johnson and G. Purvines
    1978   Inhalant Abuse among Mexican–Americans of the Southwest. In *Critical Concerns in the Field of Drug Abuse*, proceedings of Third National Drug Abuse Conference Inc, 1976, Marcel Dekker, New York.

McGrath, J.
    1986   Petrol 'Sniffing' and Lead Encephalopathy, *Medical Journal of Australia* 144(17), 221.

McGrath, A.
    1987   *Born in the Cattle: Aborigines in Cattle Country*, Allen and Unwin Australia, Sydney.

Mack, D.
    1985   *The Shepherdsons: Timber Milling in Australia 1849–1984*, Hyde Park Press, Camden Park, South Australia.

Macknight, C.C.
    1976   *The Voyage to Marege'*, Melbourne University Press, Melbourne.

McKnight, D.
    1986   Fighting in an Australian Aboriginal Supercamp. In D. Riches (ed), *The Anthropology of Violence*, Basil Blackwell, Oxford.

McMichael, A., P. Baghurst, N. Wigg, G. Vimpani, E. Robertson and R. Roberts
    1988   Port Pirie Cohort Study: Environmental Exposure to Lead and Children's Abilities at the Age of Four Years, *New England Journal of Medicine* 319(25), 468–75.

Maddock, K.
    1984   Aboriginal Customary Law. In P. Hanks and B. Keon-Cohen (eds), *Aborigines and the Law: Essays in Memory of Elizabeth Eggleston*, George Allen and Unwin, Sydney.

Mahabir, C.
    1988   Crime in the Caribbean: Robbers, Hustlers and Warriors, *International Journal of the Sociology of Law* 16, 315–38.

Mahaffey, K.R.
    1982   Role of Nutrition in Prevention of Pediatric Lead Toxicity. In J. Chisholm Jr and D.M. O'Hara (eds), *Lead Absorption in Children:*

REFERENCES

Management, Clinical and Environmental Aspects, Urban and Schwarzenbert, Baltimore/Munich.

1985   Factors Modifying Susceptibility to Lead Toxicity. In K.R. Mahaffey (ed), *Dietary and Environmental Lead: Human Health Effects*, Elsevier Science Publication B.V.

Marshall, P. (ed)
1988   *Raparapa Kularr Martuwarra: Stories from the Fitzroy River Drovers*, Magabala Books, Broome.

Mason, G. and P. Wilson
1988   *Sport, Recreation and Crime: An Assessment of the Impact of Sport and Recreation upon Aboriginal and Non-Aboriginal Youth Offenders*, Australian Institute of Criminology, Canberra.

Mathews, J.D., M.D. Riley, L. Fejo, E. Munoz, N.R. Milus, I.D. Gardner, J. Powers, E. Ganygulpa and B.J. Gununuwawuy
1988   Effects of Heavy Usage of Kava on Physical Health: Summary of a Pilot Survey in an Aboriginal Community, *Medical Journal of Australia* June 6, 148, 548–55.

May, P.
1982   Substance Abuse and American Indians: Prevalence and Susceptibility, *International Journal of the Addictions* 17(7), 1185–209.

1987   Suicide and Self-destruction among American Indian Youth, *American Indian and Alaska Native Mental Health Research* 1(1), 52–69.

Medical Research Council
1983   *Report from the MRC Advisory Group on Lead and Neuropsychological Effects in Children: A Review of the Research*, Medical Research Council, London.

Miller, M-E. and J. Ware
1989   *Mass-Media Alcohol and Drug Campaigns: A Consideration of Relevant Issues*, National Campaign Against Drug Abuse, Monograph Series no 9, Australian Government Publishing Service, Canberra.

Mills, G.G.
1986   'Sniffing With Top Spunks': Notes on the Sociopharmacology of Solvent Inhalation By Homeless Youth, *Welfare in Australia* 6(1), 10–14.

Moore, M.
1980   Exposure to Lead in Childhood: The Persisting Effects *Nature* 283 (January), 334–35.

Moore, S.F.
1983   *Law as Process: An Anthropological Approach*, Routledge and Kegan Paul, London.

Morgan, M.
　1986　　*A Drop in a Bucket: The Mount Margaret Story*, United Aborigines' Mission, Victoria.

Morice, R.D., H. Swift and M. Brady
　1981　　*Petrol Sniffing among Aboriginal Australians: A Resource Manual*, Alcohol and Drug Foundation, Canberra.

Moosa, A. and W. Loening
　1981　　Solvent Abuse in Black Children in Natal, *South African Medical Journal* 59(15), 357-60.

Myers, F.R.
　1986　　*Pintupi Country, Pintupi Self*, Australian Institute of Aboriginal Studies, Canberra/Smithsonian Institute, Washington.

New South Wales Aboriginal Education Consultative Group
　1986　　*Survey of Drug and Alcohol Use by Aboriginal School Students in New South Wales*, 84/38.1, New South Wales Aboriginal Education Consultative Group, Sydney.

National Drug Abuse Information Centre
　1989　　*Update on Deaths Caused by Volatile Substances, 1980 to 1988*, mimeograph, Commonwealth Department of Community Services and Health, Canberra.

Nganampa Health Council
　1987　　*A Strategy for Well-Being: An Environmental and Public Health Review within the Anangu Pitjantjatjara Lands*, Nganampa Health Council Inc., South Australian Health Commission and Aboriginal Health Organisation of South Australia, Adelaide.

　1989　　*Health Report 1986/1987*, Nganampa Health Council, Alice Springs.

Northern Territory Digest
　1988　　Wildman Tames 'Em, *Northern Territory Digest*, 6-8 September.

Northern Territory Department of Health
　1982　　Preface by Mary Keller. In *Discussions on Petrol Sniffing: Report of Workshops Held in Darwin and Alice Springs*, Northern Territory Health Department, Darwin.

Northern Territory Liquor Commission
　1982　　*Report on Restricted Areas*, mimeograph, Northern Territory Liquor Commission, Darwin.

Northern Youth in Crisis Conference
　1985　　*Northern Youth in Crisis: The Challenge for Justice*, resource book of materials from the Northern Youth in Crisis Conference, Quebec, November 1985, Department of Continuing Studies, Simon Fraser University, British Columbia.

Nunn, J.A. and F.M. Martin
- 1934 Gasoline and Kerosene Poisoning in Children, *Journal of the American Medical Association* 103, 472–74.

Nurcombe, B., G.N. Bianchi, J. Money and J.E. Cawte
- 1970 A Hunger for Stimuli: The Psychosocial Background of Petrol Inhalation, *British Journal of Medical Psychology* 43, 367–74.

Nwaefuna, A.
- 1981 Anorexia Nervosa in a Developing Country, *British Journal of Psychiatry* 138, 270–71.

O'Connor, R.
- 1984 Alcohol and Contingent Drunkenness in Central Australia, *Australian Journal of Social Issues* 19(3), 173–83.
- 1988 Report on the Aboriginal Alcohol Treatment/Rehabilitation Programmes Review and Consultation, prepared for the Western Australian Alcohol and Drug Authority, Perth.

O'Dea, K., N.G. White and A.J. Sinclair
- 1988 An Investigation of Nutrition-related Risk Factors in an Isolated Aboriginal Community in Northern Australia, *Medical Journal of Australia* 148, 15 February, 177–80.

Oetting, E.R., R.W. Edwards and F. Beauvais
- 1989 *Drugs and Native-American Youth*, the Haworth Press, USA.

Palmer, K. and M. Brady
- 1991 *Diet and Dust in the Desert: An Aboriginal Community, Maralinga Lands, South Australia*, Aboriginal Studies Press, Canberra.

Pearson, G.
- 1983 *Hooligan: A History of Respectable Fears*, MacMillan, London.
- 1987 *The New Heroin Users*, Basil Blackwell, Oxford, UK.

Perkins, C.
- 1975 *A Bastard Like Me*, Ure Smith, Sydney.

Peterson, N. and J. Long
- 1986 Australian Territorial Organisation: A Band Perspective, *Oceania*, Monograph 30, University of Sydney, Sydney.

Peterson, N. and M. Tonkinson
- 1979 Cobourg Peninsula and Adjacent Islands Land Claim Report to the Northern Land Council, Darwin.

Plant, A.J.
- 1988 Aboriginal Mortality in the Northern Territory 1979–1983, Masters of Public Health thesis, University of Sydney.

Plomley, N.J.B.
: 1966 : *Friendly Mission: The Tasmanian Journals and Papers of George Augustus Robinson, 1829-1934*, Tasmanian Historical Research Association, Tasmania.

Powell, A.
: 1988 : *The Shadow's Edge: Australia's Northern War*, Melbourne University Press, Melbourne.

Press, E. and A. Done
: 1967 : Solvent Sniffing, *Pediatrics* 39(3), 451-661.

Pumariega, A.J., P. Edwards and C.B. Mitchell
: 1984 : Anorexia in Black Adolescents, *Journal of the American Academy of Child Psychiatry* 23(1), 111-14.

Reay, M.
: 1982 : Abstinence, Excess and Opportunity: Minj 1963-1980. In M. Marshall (ed), *Through a Glass Darkly: Beer and Modernization in Papua New Guinea*, Monograph 18, Institute of Applied Social and Economic Research, Boroko, Papua New Guinea.

Reid, J.
: 1983 : *Sorcerers and Healing Spirits, Continuity and Change in an Aboriginal Medical System*, Australian National University Press, Canberra.

Remington, G. and B. Hoffman
: 1984 : Gas Sniffing as a Form of Substance Abuse, *Canadian Journal of Psychiatry* 29(1), 31-35.

Riley, M., L. Collins, B. Mayaninni and J. Wanytjun
: 1989 : The Body Image of East Arnhem Aborigines. In *Menzies School of Health Research Annual Report 1988-1989*, Menzies School of Health Research, Darwin.

Rischbieth, R.H., G.N. Thompson, A. Hamilton-Bruce, G.H. Purdie and J.H. Peters
: 1987 : Acute Encephalopathy following Petrol Sniffing in Two Aboriginal Patients, *Clinical and Experimental Neurology* 23, 191-94.

Robson, J.
: 1982 : Alcoholics vs Glue Sniffers, *People* 4 May, 8-10.

Rogers, G.
: 1980 : Petrol Sniffing — A Barrier to Learning, *Pivot* (South Australian Department of Education) 6(4), 24-25.

Rowse, T.
: 1987 : 'Were You Ever Savages?': Aboriginal Insiders and Pastoralists' Patronage, *Oceania* 58(1), 81-99.
: 1988 : From Houses to Households?: The Aboriginal Development Commission and Economic Adaptation by Alice Springs Town Campers, *Social Analysis* 24, December, 50-65.

Rutter, M.
1980 Raised Lead Levels and Impaired Cognitive/Behavioural Functioning: A Review of the Evidence, *Developmental Medicine and Child Neurology* (suppl.) 22(1), 1-26.

Sackett, L.
1988 Resisting Arrests: Drinking, Development and Discipline in a Desert Community, *Social Analysis* 24, December, 66-77.

Saito, K.
1973 Electroencephalographic Studies on Petrol Intoxication: Comparison between Non-leaded and Leaded White Petrol, *British Journal of Industrial Medicine* 30, 352-58.

Sandefur, J.
1985 Aspects of the Socio-political History of Ngukurr (Roper River) and Its Effect on Language Change, *Aboriginal History* 9(2), 205-19.

Sansom, B.
1980 *The Camp at Wallaby Cross: Aboriginal Fringe-Dwellers in Darwin*, Australian Institute of Aboriginal Studies, Canberra.

Sargent, G.
1977 A Discussion Paper: Appropriate Facilities for Traditional Aboriginal Children, paper to Crime Prevention Council of Australia (Northern Territory Division) 14 September.

Schottstaedt, M. and J. Bjork
1977 Inhalant Abuse in an Indian Boarding School, *American Journal of Psychiatry* 134(11), 129-33.

Senate Select Committee on Volatile Substance Fumes
1985 Senate Select Committee on Volatile Substance Fumes (Reference: Volatile Substance Fumes), *Official Hansard Report*, Australian Government Publishing Service, Canberra.

Seshia, S.S., K.R. Rajani, R.L. Boeckx and P.N. Chow
1978 The Neurological Manifestations of Chronic Inhalation of Leaded Gasoline, *Developmental Medicine and Child Neurology* 20, 323-34.

Shkilnyk, A.M.
1985 *A Poison Stronger Than Love: The Destruction of an Ojibwa Community*, Yale University Press, New Haven and London.

Sibthorpe, B.
1988 All Our People Are Dyin': Diet and Stress in an Urban Aboriginal Community, PhD thesis, Australian National University, Canberra.

Silber, T.J.
1984 Anorexia Nervosa in Black Adolescents, *Journal of the National Medical Association* 76(1), 29-32.

Smart, R.G., E.M. Adlaf and M.S. Goodstadt
    1986   Alcohol and Other Drugs among Ontario Students: An Update, *Canadian Journal of Public Health* 77 (January–February).

Smith, A. and L. McCulloch
    1986   Petrol Sniffing: Report on a Visit to Alice Springs to See the Work of the Northern Territory Petrol Sniffing Prevention Team, Department for Community Services, Perth.

Solvent Abuse Committee
    1987   *Solvent Abuse among Children and Young Adults in God's Lake Narrows*, Solvent Abuse Committee, God's Lake Narrows, Manitoba (in conjunction with the Department of Pediatrics, University of Manitoba), Canada.

South Australian Aboriginal Customary Law Committee
    1984   Children and Authority in the North West, Aboriginal Customary Law Committee, Adelaide.

Spencer, D.J.
    1988   Transitional Alcoholism – The Australian Aboriginal Model, *Technical Information Bulletin* no 79, Australian Government Publishing Service, Canberra.

Stanley, O.
    1974   Aboriginal Communities on Cattle Stations in Central Australia, *Australian Economic Papers* 15(27), 158–70.

Stanton, J.
    1988   Mt. Margaret: Missionaries and the Aftermath. In T. Swain and D.B. Rose (eds), *Aboriginal Australians and Christian Missions*, the Australian Association for the Study of Religions at the South Australian College of Advanced Education, Sturt Campus, South Australia.

State Working Party on Petrol Sniffing
    1988   *Karnanytjarra Proud and Strong*, Health Education Syllabus K-10, State Working Party on Petrol Sniffing and Aboriginal Education Resources Unit, Perth.

Stevens, F.
    1974   *Aborigines in the Northern Territory Cattle Industry*, Australian National University Press, Canberra.

Strathern, M.
    1987   Relations without Substance. In L. Lindstrom (ed), *Drugs in Western Pacific Societies: Relations of Substance*, University Press of America, Lanham.

Stryde, W.
    1977   A Report on Gasoline Sniffing in Manitoba, Department of National Health and Welfare, and Alcoholism Foundation of Manitoba, Canada.

Sullivan, J.
   1983   *Banggaiyerri: The Story of Jack Sullivan as Told to Bruce Shaw*, Australian Institute of Aboriginal Studies, Canberra.

Sweeney, G.
   1950   Inspection and Investigation, Lee Bros. Sawmill, July 1950, Australian Archives (NT): CRS F315, item 1949/393 AIII.

   1956   Employment of Aborigines at 30th June 1956 (Excluding Missions), Report to Chief Welfare Officer 24/8/56, Department of Aboriginal Affairs file 56/293, Darwin.

Taylor, E.J. (ed)
   1988   *Dorland's Illustrated Medical Dictionary*, 27th edn, W.B. Saunders Co, Philadelphia.

Tenenbein, M., W. DeGroot and K.R. Rajani
   1984   Peripheral Neuropathy following Intentional Inhalation of Naptha Fumes, *Canadian Medical Association Journal* 131, 1 November, 1077–79.

Thiele, S.
   1982   *Yugul: An Arnhem Land Cattle Station*, North Australia Research Unit, Darwin.

Thomson, D.F.
   1939   Notes on the Smoking Pipes of North Queensland and the Northern Territory of Australia, *Man* 76, 81–91.

Thomson, N.
   1985   *Aboriginal Health: Status, Programs and Prospects*, Commonwealth of Australia, Legislative Research Service Discussion Papers, no 1, Department of the Parliamentary Library, Canberra.

Thomson, N. and P. Merrifield
   1989   *Aboriginal Health: An Annotated Bibliography*, Aboriginal Studies Press, Canberra.

Tomlinson, J.
   1975   Petrol Sniffing in the Northern Territory, *Australian Journal of Alcoholism and Drug Dependence* 2(3), 74–77.

United States Department of Health, Education and Welfare
   1978   *Come Closer Round the Fire: Using Tribal Legends, Myths, and Stories in Preventing Drug Abuse*, National Institute on Drug Abuse, Prevention Branch, Rockville, Maryland, USA.

   1978   *The United States Center for Disease Control Guidelines for Preventing Lead Poisoning in Young Children*, a statement by the Center for Disease Control, Public Health Service, USA.

Usher, P.
   1987   Choosing Your Poison: Differences of Opinion about the Destruction of a Native Community, *This Magazine* 20(5), 40–44.

Valpey, R., M. Sumi, M. Copass and G. Goble
    1978   Acute and Chronic Progressive Encephalopathy due to Gasoline Sniffing, *Neurology* May, 507–10.

Viner, R.I.
    1978   Department of Aboriginal Affairs Report, Ministerial Statement, House of Representatives, *Weekly Hansard* 22, 3442–50, Australian Government Publishing Service, Canberra.

Wallace, N.M.
    1977   Change in Spiritual and Ritual Life in Pitjantjatjara (Bidjandjadjara) Society, 1966 to 1973. In R.M. Berndt (ed), *Aborigines and Change*, Australian Institute of Aboriginal Studies, Canberra.

Wardaguga, M. and M. Dawumal
    1980   Petrol Sniffing, Aboriginal Health Workers Third Annual Conference Report, Alice Springs.

Warner, W.L.
    1969   *A Black Civilization: A Social Study of an Aboriginal Tribe*, Peter Smith, Gloucester, Massachusetts.

Watson, C., J. Fleming and K. Alexander
    1988   *A Survey of Drug Use Patterns in Northern Territory Aboriginal Communities 1986–1987*, Northern Territory Department of Health and Community Services, Darwin.

Watson, P.
    1983   This Precious Foliage: A Study of the Aboriginal Psychoactive Drug 'Pituri', *Oceania*, Monograph 26, University of Sydney, Sydney.

    1987   Drugs in Trade. In L. Lindstrom (ed), *Drugs in Western Pacific Societies: Relations of Substance*, University Press of America, Lanham.

Weibel-Orlando, J.
    1989   Hooked on Healing: Anthropologists, Alcohol and Intervention, *Human Organisation* 48(2) summer, 148–55.

Williams, N.M.
    1987   *Two Laws: Managing Disputes in a Contemporary Aboriginal Community*, Australian Institute of Aboriginal Studies, Canberra.

Worrall, J.
    1982   European Courts and Tribal Aborigines — A Statistical Collection of Dispositions from the North-west Reserve of South Australia, *Australia and New Zealand Journal of Criminology* 15, 47–55.

Wright Mills, C.
    1942   The Professional Ideology of Social Pathologists, *American Journal of Sociology* 49, 165–80.

Young, E.
  1981 *Tribal Communities in Rural Areas*, Development Studies Centre, Australian National University, Canberra.

  1984 *Outback Stores: Retail Services in North Australian Aboriginal Communities*, North Australia Research Unit, Darwin.

Young, T.J.
  1987 Inhalant Use among American Indian Youth, *Child Psychiatry and Human Development* 18(1), 36–46.

Zinberg, N.E.
  1984 *Drug, Set, and Setting: The Basis for Controlled Intoxicant Use*, Yale University Press, New Haven and London.

INDEX

NOTE: * indicates an illustration or table

Aboriginal Benefits Trust Account 177
  spending on vehicles 112
Aborigines
  see also communities
  attitude to body size 78-82
  attitude to child rearing 73-74, 189, 194
  attitude to intervention 125, 172-73
  attitude to welfare officers 131, 134-45
  Christian ministry 93, 114
  community welfare 103-04
  Councils 110-11, 176-77
  effect of citizenship rights 146
  employment as youth officers 134
  fertility rates 142-43
  vehicle ownership 149
absorption differences in individuals 61-62
Action *see* rock gospel movement
Adelaide Children's Hospital
  use of chelating agents 49
alcohol
  records of use 9-10, 12
Ali Curung community
  absence of sniffing 154-57
Alice Springs Hospital
  admission of patients 65
  management of sniffing patients 48-49
Amata community
  legislative measures 22
  occurrence of sniffing 147

American Indians
  interventions 2, 174, 180
  study of alcohol and other use 20-22, 26, 70
  suicide attempts 77
Amoonguna 147
Anangu *see* Pitjantjatjara
Anglican Church
  links with settlements 114
Angurugu community 93
  acceptance of sniffing 34
  Christian influence 114
  rock gospel 116
anorexia and sniffing 78-82
areas of prevalence 13, 29-33
Arnhem Land community 60-61, 157-59*
  indulgence of children 73
  process of learning 84
  rise of gangs 88-94
  successes in curbing sniffing 157
Aurukun community
  absence of sniffing 34
Australian Institute of Petroleum
  levels of lead in petrol 66
  submission to Senate Select Committee 39-40
autonomy statements 69-97, 192

Balamumu
  arrival at Numbulwar 144
Balgo community 34
  absence of sniffing 156-57
Bathurst Island community 60

Borroloola community
  absence of sniffing 34
  social mores 186-87
bowsers with cages 13*
Brazil
  study of solvent users 27
Broome community 34
Bulla Camp
  treatment of sniffing 157
Bungalow 147
  occurrence of sniffing 146

Canada
  occurrence of petrol sniffing 19, 22-25
cattle industry
  effects of industry association 164, 183-90
chelation therapy 47-52
  disadvantages 50-51
  overseas use 50
Christian influence 93, 113-21
Church Missionary Society (CMS) 114, 161
  role at Ngukurr 164-66
clinics 46-47
communities of Aborigines
  absence of sniffing 34, 154-60
  actions to prevent sniffing 160-66, 174-80
  associations 149, 156
  distribution 29-33
  welfare 103-04
Community Development Employment Program (CDEP) 133, 134
Council for Aboriginal Alcohol Program Services (CAAPS)
  interventions 175-76

criminal offences
  association with sniffing 126
Croker Island
  early reports of sniffing 141
cursing *see* taboos

deaths from sniffing 53-62*, 191
  geographical distribution 59*-61
  increase in numbers 67*
demographics 9-10*
  rise of sniffing 142, 146, 152-53*
Department of Aboriginal Affairs 134
Department of Community Services and Health
  National Drug Abuse Information Centre
    statistics on deaths 54
deviant behaviour
  accommodation in community 70
diet *see* nutrition
Doomadgee community 34
drug use
  reasons for use 1-2, 4, 14, 24-26
drunkenness
  reaction to control 75-77

effects of sniffing
  effects on family 77
  personal effects 14, 42-44
  social effects 14
Elcho Island
  study of sniffing 26-27, 142
encephalopathy
  induction by inhalation 40-44*
  use of chelating agents 48
Ernabella mission 149*
  occurrence of sniffing 147

INDEX 219

family influence 103-11*
  abrogation of responsibilities 126
  defence of sniffers 129
  role of HALT 174
fatalities see deaths
Fitzroy Crossing community 34

Galiwin'ku community 34
  early reports of sniffing 142
  gospel movement 115
  influence on Western Desert
    communities 119
gang formation 87-95*
Goulburn Island
  early reports of sniffing 141
  establishment 144
government action 7, 193
  Aboriginal attitudes 173
  access to resources 111-13, 193
  funding for cattle industry projects
    188
  misdirection of funds 101-02, 112
  WA Working Party on Petrol
    Sniffing 17
Groote Eylandt community 34, 83
  availability of alcohol 146
  learning process 86
Gunwinggu
  arrival at Maningrida 144

Halls Creek community 34
health
  effect of incarceration 126
  effect of sniffing 16
  effect on susceptibility 62-64
Healthy Aboriginal Life Team (HALT)
  interventions 17, 174
heavy metal music 87, 91, 92*
history of sniffing

Central Australia 146-50*
northern Australia 139-46*
progression 150-52
homelands movement 111-12
  absence of sniffing 174-75
hospitals
  see also individual hospitals
  chelation therapy 48-50
  role 46-47
  treatment for encephalopathy
    40-44*
hydrocarbon toxicity 39-40

incarceration
  impact on sniffing 126, 135
Indians see American Indians
interventions 193
  Aboriginal attitudes 125, 170
  abuse of vehicles 112-13
  American Indians 2
  ceremonial avenues 179-80
  community success at Ngukurr
    162-66
  compensation payments 180
  direct confrontation 132
  HALT 17
  local initiatives 132-34
  medical interventions see chelation
    therapy
  mitigating factors 3
  overseas interventions 180-83
  shame 179
  sport 101-02
  taboos 179

Jigalong community
  absence of sniffing 34
juveniles
  see also youth

offences associated with substance
abuse 127*-28*
unwarranted focus of attention 14
work camp 126-29

Kalgoorlie Hospital
treatment of sniffers 49-50
kava use 11
Kiwirrkurra community 34
Kriol language 162-64*

languages
associations 156
distribution of Central Australian
languages 155*
Kriol 162-64*
lead absorption 38-39
legislative measures against sniffing
121-29

Maningrida community
attitude to sniffing 17
availability of alcohol 144
early reports of sniffing 141, 142
evacuations from the community
64*-65*
outstations 112
population growth 144
recovery assessment 45
rock gospel 116
maps of affected areas of Australia
29-33
Marble Bar community
absence of sniffing 34
medical services
records 6
Melville Island community 60
availability of alcohol 146
early reports of sniffing 141

methodology of research 5-7
Milingimbi community 34
early reports of sniffing 141
establishment 144
rock gospel 116
mining royalties
use of funds 177-78
Mornington Island community
effects of population increase
144-45
music *see* heavy metal

National Campaign Against Drug
Abuse 72
Ngaanyatjarra
interpretation of 'fit' 47
legislative measures 121, 122
outstations 112
social restraints to sniffing 134
use of tobacco 12
Nganampa Health Council
public health review 62-63
services to Pitjantjatjara Lands 65
Ngukurr community 93
actions to prevent sniffing 160-66
attitude to taboos 179
Christian influence 114, 165
decrease in infant mortality 143
education by Aborigines 164-65
establishment 144
participation in the cattle industry
164
rock gospel 116
Northern Territory Survey of Drug
Use Patterns in Aboriginal
Communities 19
Northern Territory
aerial medical service 65

Department of Correctional
  Services
    wilderness work camp
    126-27
Nullagine community
  absence of sniffing 34
Numbulwar community 34, 93
  Christian influence 114
  family obligations 106
  rock gospel 116
Nungalinya College 93
Nunggubuyu language 105
nutrition
  effect on susceptibility 62-63
  relation to sniffing 78-82

obesity 81-82
Oenpelli community
  early reports of sniffing 141
  availability of alcohol 146
outstations *see* homelands movement
Outward Bound
  similarity to wilderness work camp
  126-27

Papua New Guinea
  alcohol use 170
  substance use 172-73
Papunya
  absence of sniffing 154
Perkins, Charles
  comments on sniffing 146
petrol sniffing
  effects of use 37-52*
  attitudes 13, 16-17, 169-73
petrol toxicity 37-52*
Pintupi community 72
  concept of family 105

Pitjantjatjara
  attitude to obesity 82
  attitude to research 5, 6
  attitude to sniffers 47, 74-75, 134
  concept of family 105
  distribution of marriage alliances
    148*
  early reports of sniffing 147
  effect of Christian revival 120
  food taboos 171
  generosity of spirit 73
  health services 65
  legislative measures 121-25
  map of lands 124*
  review of health 63
  sniffing at outstations 112
  sugar intake 81
policing 129-31, 136
  police powers 121, 123, 130
  presence in Anangu Pitjantjatjara
    Lands 125
Princess Alexandra Hospital
  treatment of sniffers 50

Ramingining community 34
  early reports of sniffing 141, 142
reasons for sniffing 14, 69-98, 150
  Canadian experience 24-26
recovery from sniffing 44-46, 95
references 195-215
regional variations in Australia
  25-35*
regional variations overseas 22-27
research
  methodology 5-7
  Yalata community 132-34
restraints to sniffing 99-102
rituals of sniffing 86-87
rock gospel movement 115-18*

Roper River *see* Ngukurr
Rose River Mission 144
Royal Commission into Aboriginal
    Deaths in Custody
    effect on apprehension of sniffers
        125
Royal Darwin Hospital
    evacuations of sniffers 64–65
    use of chelating agents 48
Royal Flying Doctor Service (RFDS)
    attitude to sniffers 46–47
    policy in WA 66

sanctions *see* restraints
Senate Select Committee into
    Volatile Substance Fumes 12
        comments by Charles Perkins 146
        findings 3, 14, 16
            deaths 54
        Institute of Petroleum submission
            39–40
set 3–5
setting 3–5, 131, 135, 192, 194
social influences 82–87, 102–11,
    134–36, 169–80
South Australia
    Drug and Alcohol Services Council
        133
sporting facilities
    use and misuse 101–02, 177–78
statistics 27–33, 128–29
    deaths from sniffing 53–61*
    inadequacies of information 6, 44
substance use
    Canadian findings 23–26
    learning process 83–87
    overview 9–18
summary 7

susceptibility to effects of sniffing
    62–64

taboos 91
    effect on resistance to substance
        abuse 171, 179
tobacco 10–11, 12
    analgesic use 11
toxicity of petrol 37–52*

Umbakumba community
    methods to prevent sniffing 158–60
unemployment
    psychological effects 189
United Aborigines' Mission 119–20

videos
    influence in Arnhem Land 89

Warburton community
    treatment of fits 47
welfare officers
    effect on sniffing 134–35
    role 131–32
Western Australia
    evacuation of sniffers 66
    levels of lead in petrol 66
    State Working Party on Petrol
        Sniffing 113, 129
wilderness work camp 126–29
Wildman River
    camp for juvenile offenders
        127–29, 135
Wiluna community
    absence of sniffing 34
    behaviour when drunk 75

Yalata homeland centre 112
    research 132–34

Yirrkala community
  rock gospel 116
Yolngu
  Christian revival 114
youth
  attitude to Christian ethics 176–77
  influence of associates 130–31
  lack of prestige 179
  offences associated with substance abuse 127*–28*
  rock gospel movement 115
  role models 153–54
  social needs 82–83, 94
  statistics on deaths 58
  use of inhalants 11–12, 22
Yuendumu community 34
  absence of sniffing 154
  growth rate 143